ENDOCRINOLOGY RESEARCH AND CLIN

HYPOTHYROIDISM

DIAGNOSIS AND SCREENING, GENETIC INFLUENCES AND TREATMENT OPTIONS

ENDOCRINOLOGY RESEARCH AND CLINICAL DEVELOPMENTS

Additional books in this series can be found on Nova's website under the Series tab.

Additional e-books in this series can be found on Nova's website under the e-book tab.

ENDOCRINOLOGY RESEARCH AND CLINICAL DEVELOPMENTS

HYPOTHYROIDISM

DIAGNOSIS AND SCREENING, GENETIC INFLUENCES AND TREATMENT OPTIONS

ASHLEY O'NEILL
AND
MASON R. QUINN
EDITORS

New York

For permission to use material from this book please contact us:
Telephone 631-231-7269; Fax 631-231-8175
Web Site: http://www.novapublishers.com

Library of Congress Cataloging-in-Publication Data

ISBN: 978-1-62618-872-3

Library of Congress Control Number: 2013938112

Published by Nova Science Publishers, Inc. † New York

Contents

Preface

Hypothyroidism is a state in which the thyroid gland does not make enough thyroid hormone. Iodine deficiency is often cited as the most common cause of hypothyroidism worldwide but it can be caused by many other factors. It can result from the lack of a thyroid gland or from iodine-131 treatment, and can also be associated with increased stress. In this book, the authors present current research in the study of the diagnosis and screening, genetic influences and treatment options for hypothyroidism. Topics include low T3 syndrome and subclinical hypothyroidism; age-based TSH levels in hypothyroidism treatment; overt hypothyroidism, subclinical hypothyroidism and isolated hypothyroxinemia during pregnancy; and thyroid hypofunction in pregnancy.

Chapter I – The hormones triiodothyronine (T_3) and tetraiodothyronine (T_4), produced by the thyroid gland, are important to maintain adequate levels of energy in human body and in particular, at the cellullar level are essential in maintaining the initial level of phospholipids in cell membranes and fatty acids composition of the lipids; in particular T_3 plays a critical role in lipid metabolism by regulating genes involved in lipogenesis and lipolysis. Respiratory chain is regulated by thyroid hormones (TH). In addition to their metabolic role, it is also well known that TH have important tissutal effects: they have inotropic and chronotropic positive effect, have a role in the bone's turn-over, have a stimulating effect on intestinal peristalsis and in both sexes influence sexual development and reproductive function. Hypothyroidism is an endocrine disorder resulting from deficiency of TH or its effects on peripheral tissues and it is clear that it can result in both metabolic and tissutal alterations of various degrees. However, while hypothyroidism is a condition well known, there are other conditions not so well characterized that often create problems of therapeutic management: subclinical hypothyroidism (a serum thyroid stimulating hormone (TSH) above the defined upper limit of the reference range, with a serum free thyroxine (fT_4) within the reference range, with little or no clinical features) and the so called "non thyroidal illness syndrome" (NTIS) (a low T_3 state described in a variety of clinical situations, such as starvation, sepsis, surgery, trauma, heart failure, respiratory failure and other severe illness, considered an adaptive response rather than true hypothyroidism). The situation of NTIS is very complex: data in literature support the hypothesis of a biochemical, rather than clinical, benefit of therapy with T_3 administration. However, data of the authors' group, performed in patients with chronic obstructive pulmonary disease, suggest an hypothyroidism at tissue level, since metabolic data are similar to those of patients with manifested hypothyroidism (plasma elevation of the respiratory chain component Coenzyme Q_{10} and reduced plasma antioxidant capacity, suggesting increased oxidative stress in such a condition). Conflicting data are similarly reported in subclinical hypothyroidism: it can be associated with luteal deficiency and infertility in women, who benefit from replacement therapy.

Chapter II – The goal of hypothyroidism treatment is restoration of the euthyroid state in all the tissues. Monitoring the adequacy of levothyroxine therapy is easily done by measuring the serum thyrotropin (TSH) levels. This measurement should be within the normal range. The National Health and Nutrition Examinations Survey (NHANES) sampling attempts to represent the U.S. population. Data from NHANES indicates that in population with iodine sufficiency, the serum TSH levels increase with age. Furthermore, in people with no clinical or biochemical experience of thyroid disease, no change has been observed in free thyroxine (FT4) concentrations. Other results from cross-sectional studies have also found an increase in TSH with age in populations free of thyroid disease. Additionally the raised of TSH observed in people with exceptional longevity suggests that the change of thyroid axis could be protective. Thus, it seems that there is a progressive shift in the serum TSH distribution curve toward higher TSH values with increasing age. Based on these results, some researchers recommend the adoption of age-specific reference ranges for TSH, however this remains a matter of debate. This chapter is aimed to review medical research supporting the use of age- specific TSH reference ranges and subsequently an age-related TSH target to treat hypothyroidism.

Chapter III – Thyroid dysfunction is common during gestation. The prevalence of hypothyroidism during pregnancy is estimated to be 0.3-0.5%

for overt hypothyroidism (OH) and 2-3% for subclinical hypothyroidism (SCH). The prevalence of isolated hypothyroxinemia is 1-2% in sufficient iodine intake regions. Chronic autoimmune thyroiditis is the main cause of hypothyroidism during pregnancy, apart from iode deficiency. Reference ranges for thyroid function tests differ in healthy pregnant women from those of healthy non pregnant women. A TSH of 2.5 mIU/l is now accepted as the upper limit of normal for TSH in the first trimester. OH is defined as an elevated TSH (>2.5 mIU/l) in conjunction with a decreased free T4 (FT4) concentration. Women with TSH levels of 10.0 mIU/l or above, irrespective of their FT4 levels are also considered to have OH. SCH is defined as a serum TSH between 2.5 and 10.0 mIU/l with a normal FT4 concentration. Isolated hypothyroxinemia is defined as a normal maternal TSH concentration in conjunction with FT4 concentrations in the lower 5th or 10th percentile of the reference range. It is now well established that OH is associated with an increased risk of adverse pregnancy complications, as well as detrimental effects upon fetal neurocognitive development. However, data regarding SCH and maternal isolated hypothyroxinemia are controversial. In the past several years, there has been considerable discussion about whether all pregnant women should be screened in order to identify and treat thyroid dysfunction. To date there are not enough data for or against universal screening. In their recent guidelines, the American Thyroid Association and the Endocrine Society recommend prenatal measurement of serum TSH in women at high risk for thyroid illness on the basis of their medical history, physical exam, or prior chemical data. Women with preexisting hypothyroidism will need to increase their prepregnancy dose of thyroxine to maintain a normal thyroid function. In a newly diagnosed hypothyroid patient, a full replacement thyroxine dose should be instituted immediately and thyroxine dosage adjusted on the base of results of thyroid function tests. Serum FT4 level should be at the upper end of normal range for each trimester of pregnancy, serum TSH level should be < 2.5 mIU/L in the first trimester or 3 mIU/l in the second and third trimesters. Since maternal morbidity as well as prenatal morbidity and consequences on the neuropsychological development of the child have been reported in subclinical hypothyroidism, most guidelines recommend thyroxine replacement in women with subclinical hypothyroidism. Management of isolated hypothyroxinemia during pregnancy is controversial and requires further study.

Chapter IV – Thyroid hypofunction in pregnancy is associated with either overt or subclinical hypothyroidism. Many studies reported a link between hypothyroidism and infertility as well as with a high rate of spontaneous miscarriages. These pregnancies are though very precious for the patients. Woman of childbearing age must then be aware of the necessity of an adapted treatment and of a close monitoring in case of a possible pregnancy as well as of risks for herself and for the newborn child. Once the diagnosis is done, the treatment with oral LT4 is very simple. The monitoring will be made every 2 months (at least) to adapt the treatment to the objectives of TSH which are different from the common population. After a short case report of 15 women of childbearing age followed for hypothyroidism from January to February 2009, the authors decided to educate all the women of childbearing age because even treated appropriately with oral LT4, they were not sensitized to the necessity of increasing the dose and the follow up in case of pregnancy! We believe that preconceptional counseling is very important and could improve the management of these very precious pregnancies. In practice, if the hypothyroidism is known, and if a pregnancy is wished, it is necessary to insure a hormonal balance before the conception. We advise to tell the patient they should increase their dose of oral LT4 by 25% to 30%.

In: Hypothyroidism
Editors: A. O'Neill and M. R. Quinn
ISBN: 978-1-62618-872-3

Chapter I

Evidence of Tissue Hypothyroidism: The Low T_3 Syndrome and Subclinical Hypothyroidism

A. Mancini, S. Raimondo, C. Di Segni, M. Persano, A. Saporosi and E. Giacchi

Department of Internal Medicine, Division of Endocrinology,
Centre for Study and Research on Natural Fertility Regulation,
Catholic University of the Sacred Heart, Rome, Italy

Abstract

The hormones triiodothyronine (T_3) and tetraiodothyronine (T_4), produced by the thyroid gland, are important to maintain adequate levels of energy in human body and in particular, at the cellullar level are essential in maintaining the initial level of phospholipids in cell membranes and fatty acids composition of the lipids; in particular T_3 plays a critical role in lipid metabolism by regulating genes involved in lipogenesis and lipolysis. Respiratory chain is regulated by thyroid hormones (TH).

In addition to their metabolic role, it is also well known that TH have important tissutal effects: they have inotropic and chronotropic positive effect, have a role in the bone's turn-over, have a stimulating effect on intestinal peristalsis and in both sexes influence sexual development and reproductive function.

Hypothyroidism is an endocrine disorder resulting from deficiency of TH or its effects on peripheral tissues and it is clear that it can result in both metabolic and tissutal alterations of various degrees. However, while hypothyroidism is a condition well known, there are other conditions not so well characterized that often create problems of therapeutic management: subclinical hypothyroidism (a serum thyroid stimulating hormone (TSH) above the defined upper limit of the reference range, with a serum free thyroxine (fT_4) within the reference range, with little or no clinical features) and the so called "non thyroidal illness syndrome" (NTIS) (a low T_3 state described in a variety of clinical situations, such as starvation, sepsis, surgery, trauma, heart failure, respiratory failure and other severe illness, considered an adaptive response rather than true hypothyroidism). The situation of NTIS is very complex: data in literature support the hypothesis of a biochemical, rather than clinical, benefit of therapy with T_3 administration. However, data of our group, performed in patients with chronic obstructive pulmonary disease, suggest an hypothyroidism at tissue level, since metabolic data are similar to those of patients with manifested hypothyroidism (plasma elevation of the respiratory chain component Coenzyme Q_{10} and reduced plasma antioxidant capacity, suggesting increased oxidative stress in such a condition).

Conflicting data are similarly reported in subclinical hypothyroidism: it can be associated with luteal deficiency and infertility in women, who benefit from replacement therapy.

Introduction

The hormones triiodothyronine (T_3) and tetraiodothyronine (T_4), produced by the thyroid gland, are important to maintain adequate levels of energy in human body and in particular, at the cellullar level, are essential in maintaining the initial level of phospholipids in cell membranes and fatty acids composition of the lipids; especially T_3 plays a critical role in lipid metabolism by regulating genes involved in lipogenesis and lipolysis [1]. Respiratory chain is regulated by thyroid hormones (TH) [2].

In addition to their metabolic role, it is also well known that TH have important tissutal effects: they have inotropic and chronotropic positive effect, have a role in the bone's turn-over, have a stimulating effect on intestinal peristalsis and in both sexes influence sexual development and reproductive function [3].

Hypothyroidism is an endocrine disorder resulting from deficiency of TH or its effects on peripheral tissues and it is clear that it can result in both metabolic and tissutal alterations of various degrees such as gain of weight, weakness, bradycardia, menstrual disturbances and interference with male fertility, dyslipidemia, depressed mood, constipation and so on.

Hypothyrodism, in particular the thyroid hormone deficiency due to abnormality in the thyroid gland (primary hypothyroidism), is the most common endocrine disease. The prevalence of hypothyroidism in the general population ranges from 3.8%–4.6% [4-7] and it most affects aging women [8]. Autoimmune thyroiditis is the most common cause of primary hypothyrodism, even if, in many parts of the world, iodine deficiency is still an important cause; other important and very common cause of hypothyroidism are thyroidectomy, radioiodine therapy, and drugs such as amiodarone, lithium, thionamide, iodine, interferon, sunitinib, rifampicin, and thalidomide [9].

Congenital hypothyroidism, defined as thyroid hormone deficiency present at birth, affects about one in 2000-4000 newborns and is the commonest congenital endocrinopathy [10]. It is due, in most cases, by alterations in the embryogenesis of the thyroid gland like the absence of the gland itself (agenesis), hypoplasia, or the presence of thyroid sketches in ectopic sites (ectopia), which are generally insufficient to ensure a normal secretion of thyroid hormones. More rarely, the congenital hypothyroidism is caused by a genetically determined deficiency of enzymes responsible for the synthesis of thyroid hormones. Damage due to prolonged lack of thyroid hormones are multiple and disseminated to all organs and systems. In particular, lesions of the central nervous system lead to severe mental retardation so it is therefore of primary importance timely diagnosis (which is more often achieved through screening programs) and the immediate start of replacement therapy with thyroxine.

The thyroid gland is regulated by the pituitary gland and the hypothalamus, so thyroid disorders may result not only from defects in the thyroid itself but also from the disruption of the control system in these other organs (secondary hypothyroidism). A failure of the pituitary gland to secrete thyroid stimulating hormone (TSH), usually caused by a tumor in the region of the pituitary, due to a lack of stimulation of the thyroid to produce T_3 and T_4, resulting in hypothyroidism.

Both in primary and secondary hypothyroidism signs and symptoms were consistent. Early symptoms includes weakness, fatigue, cold intolerance, constipation, weight gain, depression, joint or muscle pain, brittle fingernails, coarseness, thinning of hair; instead late symptoms: slow speech, dry and flaky skin, thickening of the skin, puffy face, hands, and feet, decreased hearing, thinning of eyebrows, menstrual disorders and interference with male fertility, depressed mood [11].

Hypothyroidism has a profound impact on metabolism. One of the elements that characterizes hypothyroidism is an increased fasting plasma cholesterol and triglyceride levels [12]. Thyroid hormone induces the hepatic expression of hydroxymethylglutaryl coenzyme A reductase, which results in increased cholesterol synthesis [13]. The lipid pattern is characterized by elevation in lipoprotein a [Lp(a)], levels [14] (a low-density lipoprotein (LDL)- like particle synthesized by the liver that has been reported to promote thrombosis, inflammation and foam cell formation) [15] and in total cholesterol and low-density lipoprotein cholesterol (LDL-C) caused by changes in the synthesis, metabolism, and mobilization of lipids. Indeed hepatic cholesterol synthesis is decreased, but TH also increases, in liver and in other tissues, the cellular expression of LDL-C receptors [16].

Patients with hypothyroidism also have elevated levels of high-density lipoprotein cholesterol (HDL-C), primarily connected to increased concentration of cholesterol and phospholipid-enriched HDL-2 particles [16].

A decreased HDL2 catabolism and cholesteryl ester transfer protein activity has been observed. This decrease leads to a reduced transfer of cholesteryl esters from HDL to very-low-density lipoprotein (VLDL), thus increasing HDL-C levels [17].

However, while hypothyroidism is a condition well known, there are other conditions not so well characterized that often create problems of therapeutic management: the so called "non thyroidal illness syndrome" (NTIS) (a low T_3 state described in a variety of clinical situations, such as starvation, sepsis, surgery, trauma, heart failure, respiratory failure and other severe illness, considered an adaptive response rather than true hypothyroidism) and subclinical hypothyroidism.

Low-T_3 syndrome is a condition characterized by a reduced peripheral conversion from T_4 to T_3 in presence of normal thyroid hormone secretion [18,19].

The NTIS occurs in many acute conditions and the most common are: critical illness, starvation, eating disorders. For example during starvation (especially carbohydrate deprivation) and non-thyroid illness, deiodination of T_4 to T_3 is rapidly inhibited, causing the low-T_3 syndrome. An important data is that as much the illness is severe, more is complex the syndrome with low

T_3 and T_4. In critical illness, even in patients without previous diagnosis of intrinsic thyroid disease, several abnormalities in thyroid hormone (TH) secretion, metabolism and action have been observed and these changes have been defined overall NTIS [18]; this term is now largely employed, in the place of "euthyroid sick syndrome" [20-22] or "low-T_3 syndrome", due to the most common abnormality, a decreased level of serum total T_3, which can be within 2 hours after the onset of severe physical stress [23-25]. However, T_3 lowering is only one of the endocrine elements described is such a situation; therefore the term NTIS seems to be more appropriate, also strengthening its extrathyroidal source.

NTIS has been depicted in about 70% of hospitalized patients for different diseases [26-28] but there is a strong correlation also between the severity of morbidity and outcome in patients studied in intensive care unit (ICU) and the alteration in thyroid function [29-30]. At any rate the hormonal response is different in acute and chronic phase: in the first phase the alteration predominate in peripheral metabolism of TH, while in the latter central mechanisms controlling thyroid secretion progressively arise [31,32].

In NTIS there is no clear evidence of tissue hypothyroidism, so most of authors consider this condition as an adaptative response, that does not usually require a thyroid replacement therapy, but this topic is still debated, since indirect signs of true hypothyroidism at tissue levels have been showed [33]. The question is still open and different reviews have been published on this topic [18, 34-38] but there is still no an unanimous agreement on the procedure to follow.

Very recently different molecular mechanism have been shown to gain insight the complex situation of NTIS and in particular we have been underlined the role of intracellular oxidative stress (OS).

Another peculiar situation is subclinical hypothyroidism, a serum TSH above the defined upper limit of the reference range, with a serum fT_4 within the reference range, with little or no clinical features [39].

Indexes of Tissue Hypothyroidism

In both the conditions above defined, a number of paper was directed to search for indexes of tissue hypothyroidism, studying the pattern of serological parameters influenced by TH, such as angiotensin-converting enzyme (ACE), sex hormone binding globulin (SHBG) and osteocalcin (OC).

ACE levels have been evaluated as an index of thyroid hormone action in severe systemic illness [40]: they were elevated in hyperthyroid patients and depressed in hypothyroid patients. Compared with normal controls, patients in an intensive care unit with free thyroxine index greater than 5.0 had normal ACE levels, but patients with a free thyroxine index less than 5.0 had ACE levels significantly lower than the normal and hypothyroid groups. A group of patients in an intensive care unit with alcoholic liver disease (known to elevate ACE) and a low free thyroxine index had depressed ACE levels. A strong correlation was seen in the combined groups of all patients studied between levels of ACE and a free thyroxine index or free T_3 index.

Another parameter influenced by thyroid hormones is sex-hormone binding globulin (SHBG); due to its role in reproductive medicine and the relationships between thyroid and gonads, it appeared to be useful to investigate its possible role as index of thyroid function [41]. An increase in SHBG has been a feature consistently associated with thyrotoxicosis, leading to increased circulating levels of total testosterone and reduction in testosterone metabolic clearance rate [42-43]. On the contrary primary hypothyroidism results in a decrease in SHBG and total testosterone concentrations, and free testosterone concentrations are reduced in approximately 60% of males with hypothyroidism. In a prospective study of 10 men with primary hypothyroidism, plasma free testosterone levels were low and increased after the onset of levothyroxine (LT4) therapy [44]. It has been shown that TH administration to hypothyroid men induces a rise in both SHBG and total serum testosterone [45]. This field is very complex due to the relationships between thyroid and reproduction: boys with congenital hypothyroidism (CH) diagnosed and treated soon after birth have normal sexual development and adult height, indicating that CH does not produce long-term detrimental effects on gonadal function [46]. Although prolactin (PRL) elevation is the common link between primary hypothyroidism and gonadal dysfunction in females, instead males with primary hypothyroidism seldom exhibit elevated serum PRL concentrations, except those with long-standing and severe hypothyroidism. Severe primary hypothyroidism results in pituitary tumors in men with hyperprolactinemia and hypogonadotropic hypogonadism. Replacement therapy with TH reverses all of these abnormalities [47-49].

To test the hypothesis that patients with systemic nonthyroidal illness (NTI) and impaired thyroid hormone metabolism most commonly present with the low T_3 or low T_4 syndrome are in an euthyroid status at the tissue level, sex hormone-binding globulin (SHBG) and osteocalcin (OC) were evaluated as parameters for thyroid hormone availability to liver and bone [50]. Serum SHBG and OC concentrations were measured in 61 severely ill patients with decreased serum levels of either T_3 alone or both T_3 and free T_4. None of the patients had primary thyroid disorder indicated by regular thyroid sonomorphology and normal basal TSH concentrations. Data were compared with values obtained from age- and sex-matched controls without impairment of thyroid hormone physiology. However, in this study, SHBG and OC do not differ significantly between NTI patients with low T_3 or low T_4 syndrome and controls, and no significant relationship was found between thyroid hormone parameters and SHBG or OC, respectively, therefore in partial contradiction to the results of previous studies using alternative serum parameters for assessment of peripheral thyroid hormone action (e.g. angiotensin-converting enzyme), as above reported. The authors conclude that the term euthyroid sick syndrome applied for the condition of systemic NTI associated with reduced circulating thyroid hormone concentrations appears to be appropriate at the level of hepatocytes and osteoblasts. Due to the tissue specificity of the biochemical serum markers, conflicting results may be explained by organ-specific differences in local thyroid hormone exposure. In case of doubt, SHBG and OC determinations may help specify peripheral thyrometabolic status in NTI.

Among other parameters evaluated to investigate peripheral TH effect we can also mention fibronectin and precollagen-peptide I and III [51], in fact TH have a profound effect on bone formation and reabsorption, interacting with local factors [52].

It is useful to precise some aspects about the Coenzyme Q_{10} (CoQ_{10}), also called ubiquinone because of its ubiquitous diffusion in organisms and tissues. It is a key component of the mitochondrial oxidative phosphorylation chain as link between flavoproteins and cytochroms in the inner mitochondrial membrane. It has also many other functions, first of all a powerful antioxidant activity, and new roles in different cellular functions are coming out in last times, because this molecule can partecipate in oxido-reductive reactions not only in mitochondria, but also in lysosomial, in Golgi apparatus and plasmatic membranes [53], even contributing to membrane fluidity. Moreover CoQ_{10} can take part in many aspects of the oxido-reductive control of the cellular signalling origin and transmission; in fact the auto-oxidation of semi-quinon, formed in various membranes during the electronic transportation, can be a primary source for the H_2O_2 generation, which activates some transcription factors, as NFkB, to induce gene expression [54]. It is also possible that ROS generation could suppress other genes.

CoQ_{10} levels can be measured by HPLC, with a method standardized by the International CoQ_{10} Association [55]. Furthermore, electrochemical detection allows to assay even the reduced (ubiquinol) and oxidized (ubiquinone) forms of CoQ_{10} [56].

In a previous study, we found a significant inverse correlation between thyroid hormones and plasma CoQ_{10} [57]. This correlation was further confirmed in other studies [58] and in a larger group of patients. Fig. 1 shows a very strong correlation considering a population composed of 27 hyperthyroid patients (3 males and 24 females, aged 18-58 yrs), 24 euthyroid subjects (24 controls, 4 males and 20 females, aged 25-64 yrs) and 27 hypothyroid patients (12 males and 15 females, aged 27-68 yrs, affected by primary or secondary hypothyroidism). Values of CoQ_{10} in hyperthyroid patients are among the lowest reported in different human diseases. The reasons for this phenomenon include: decreased synthesis related to competition for tyrosine, which is a common substrate for CoQ_{10} and thyroxine synthesis, even if this hypothesis is disconfirmed by experimental data in animals; increased CoQ_{10} utilization, due to the increased metabolic demand; increased degradation; decreased levels of carriers in serum, since it is demonstrated that release of VLDL from liver is decreased in hyperthyroidism. Symmetrical mechanisms can be invoked to explain high CoQ_{10} levels in hypothyroid patients. Pharmacological treatment with metimazole restored normal values of thyroid hormones.

To further investigate tissue *vs* plasma compartment we also tested a group of patients who underwent total thyroidectomy for papillary carcinoma and multinodular goiter, allowing to obtain, from each patient, normal and pathological tissue samples. We found that patients with non toxic multinodular goiter exhibited low CoQ_{10} values in pathological areas, probably related to colloid accumulation; on the contrary, in active proliferating tissues (toxic goiter or neoplasia) CoQ_{10} concentrations were greater than in unaffected areas [59]. These data indicated increased CoQ_{10} synthesis related to increased metabolic demand.

This correlation could cover diagnostic usefulness in those clinical conditions characterized by uncoupling of thyroid hormone levels and metabolic status, like amiodarone-induced thyroid dysfunction [57] and inappropriate TSH secretion [60]. We tested a group of patients with low-T_3 syndrome due to chronic obstructive pulmonary disease: again CoQ_{10} was higher in low-T_3 syndrome than in patients with the same disease and normal T_3 levels, suggesting that real hypothyroidism could be present in this clinical situation [61].

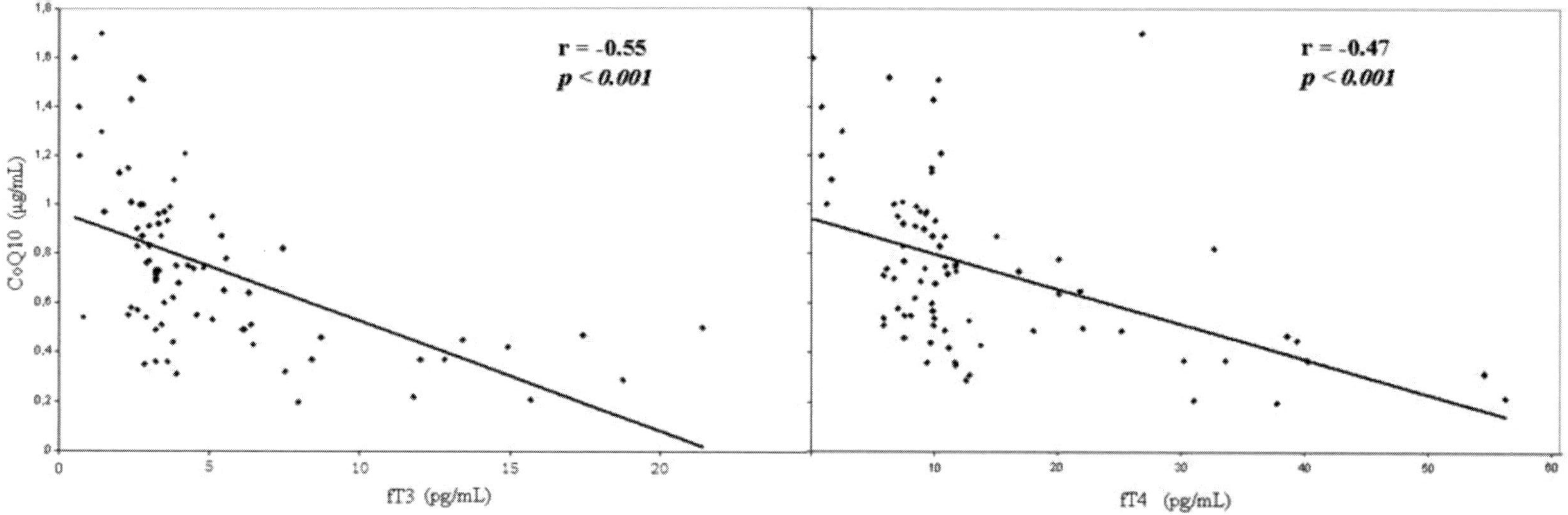

Figure 1. Scatter plots showing the strong linear correlations between Coenzyme Q_{10} and free-T_3 or free-T_4 levels in a sample composed by hyper- normo- and hypo-thyroid patients (r = Pearson coefficient) (from Mancini et al., J Endocrinol Invest, 2010, with permission).

CoQ10, other than metabolic role, has powerful antoxidant properties, due to the recycle from ubiquinol to ubiquinone form. Therefore, it appeared useful to evaluate its pattern in relation to other antioxidant. Recently a lot of methods have been developed in order to measure the total antioxidant status in biological fluids. Total antioxidant capacity (TAC) is a measurement of the non-enzymatic antioxidants, that are primarily extracellular (ascorbate, urates, albumin, tocopherol and glutathione). They are "chain-breaking" molecules able to block the propagation chain of lipid peroxidation and to prevent the amplification of radical generation and the subsequent biochemical damage. Differently by enzymes, they are consumed at the moment in which they act and this fact could explain the reduction in their levels in biological fluids producing ROS (for example, the high levels of ROS and a low TAC in the seminal fluid of infertile males suggests oxidative stress is associated to a variety of etiologies of male infertility) [62].

The dosage of TAC is considered a better index of the total antioxidant status of a biological sample than the measurement of one or more specific antioxidant, that could not carefully reflect the combined effect of the various antioxidant and their "collaboration" during the oxidative stress.

The method of Rice and Evans [63] consists in TAC evaluation by using the system metmyoglobin-H_2O_2, as source of radicals, in presence of the chromogenous 2,2^I-azinobis-(3-ethylbenzothiazoline-6-sulphonate), the radical form of which is spectroscopically detectable after a latency time (Lag) due, and therefore proportional to the antioxidant content; we have applied it, with some modifications [64], to different models of endocrine disorders.

We studied a group of hyperthyroid patients, measuring TAC and we found values similar to those of controls; nevertheless, despite higher CoQ_{10} values, TAC remained low, suggesting that oxidative stress can induce a consumption of antioxidants, but the metabolic role of CoQ_{10} is prevalent [65].

The results could be different in secondary hypothyroidism, in which the defect can be associated with multiple pituitary deficiencies, also affecting both TAC and CoQ_{10}. For instance, a rationale for studying CoQ_{10} in pituitary-adrenal disease is the common biosynthetic pathway of cholesterol and ubiquinone; we previously showed that CoQ_{10} levels were reduced in isolated hypoadrenalism. Other data indicate that secretion of adrenal hormones is in some way related to CoQ_{10} levels, both in augmented and reduced conditions [66]. However in secondary hypoadrenalism, some other pituitary dependent axes can be affected. Therefore we compared patients with post-surgical isolated hypoadrenalism with those who presented also hypothyroidism. Since thyroid hormones have an important role in modulating CoQ_{10} levels and metabolism, when coexistent, thyroid deficiency seems to play a prevalent role with respect to adrenal deficiency.

Similarly, to investigate the role of gonadal steroids in systemic antioxidant regulation, we determined plasma CoQ_{10} and TAC in post-surgical hypopituitaric patients. CoQ_{10} levels were significantly lower in isolated hypogonadism than in normogonadism. Testosterone treatment induced a significant change both in CoQ_{10} level and TAC. CoQ_{10} and TAC values significantly correlated, suggesting an inter-relationship between different antioxidants [67]. Our data suggest that hypogonadism could represent a condition of oxidative stress, in turn related with augmented cardiovascular risk. Once again, when hypogonadism was associated to hypothyroidism, the effect of the latter was prevalent.

Therefore, as a whole, experimental data indicate that CoQ10 levels can be considered a reliable index of thyroid action at tissue level.

Clinical Observations in NTIS

We recently reviewed clinical studies in NTIS and their physiopatological and therapeutic implications [19]. A low T_3 state has been described in a variety of clinical situations, such as starvation [68], sepsis [69], surgery [70], trauma [71], myocardial infarction and heart failure [72, 73], cardiopulmonary bypass [74], respiratory failure [75], bone marrow transplantation [76], other severe illness [77]. In a very recent paper it was demonstrated that in unselected ICU patients, free T_3 (fT_3) was the most powerful and the only independent predictor of ICU mortality, and when it was added to APACHE II score had a prognostic improving value [78]. Even a retrospective study in a large group of patients treated with mechanical ventilation (MV) confirmed that NTIS represent a risk factor for prolonged MV [79].

TH influence cardiac function with different mechanisms: inotropic and chronotropic positive effect via nuclear and non-nuclear pathways in cardiomyocytes, increase in cardiac contractility through augmented tissue oxygen delivery and consumption; decrease in systemic vascular resistance, through direct TH action on vascular smooth muscle cells; other endocrine effects are exerted on renin-angiotensin-aldosterone axis and on erythropoietin secretion [37, 80]. Considering the very important role in cardiac function, cardiac patients have been studied under this profile. It is known that patients with heart failure have low T_3 serum concentrations, which correlate with cardiac function [80].

One of the early studies was performed in patients after acute myocardial infarction; a notable and prolonged decrease of total T_3 (TT_3) and fT_3 was described, while TT_4 but not fT_4 showed a transient decrease; thyroxine binding globulin (TBG) levels remained unchanged, while thyroxine binding prealbumin (TBPA) and albumin exhibited a prolonged fall. TSH, despite low T_3, did not increase, remaining inappropriately low [81]. In this sense, the increase of TSH was shown to be correlated with a good prognosis [82], instead NTIS has been overall considered a strong predictor of death and it is directly correlated with a poor prognosis of cardiac patients, especially those admitted in a cardiology department [81]. In fact the low T_3 serum concencentration is directly correlated with cardiac function. In advanced heart failure, a low fT_3 index/reverse T_3 ratio was associated with higher right atrial pulmonary artery and pulmonary capillary wedge and lower ejection fraction [73].

TH are implicated in metabolic function of myocardial cells; they have been shown to inversely correlate with Coenzyme Q_{10} (CoQ_{10}), a component of mitochondrial respiratory chain, also endowed with powerful antioxidant properties, as above described [57]. Our group studied patients after major heart surgery and showed low T_3 levels joint to signs of tissue hypothyroidism (elevated CoQ_{10} levels, despite the fact that cardiac disease are well known to be associated with low CoQ) [60].

Unlike of cardiac patients, the pulmonary disorders have not been so extensively studied [83-85]. In the just cited paper, low T_3 state was again considered a predictor of outcome in respiratory failure [75]. Among chronic conditions, no conclusive data are reported on chronic obstructive pulmonary disease (COPD), as reported in a recent review [86]. In COPD has not been reported an evident alteration in thyroid function [87], although patients with severe hypoxemia showed a strong positive correlation between total T_3/total T_4 ratio (TT_3/TT_4) and PaO_2 [88]. In stable COPD has been reported an increased fT_3 concentrations, with a positive association to $PaCO_2$ [86], while others reported, in patients with severe hypoxemia, lower total T_3, fT_3 and TT_3/TT_4 ratios [89]. Low Forced Espiratory Volume at 1st second (FEV_1) is associated with low basal and stimulated levels of thyroid stimulating hormone (TSH) [90], but the real impact of hypoxemia on TSH response to exogenous thyrotropin releasing hormone (TRH) is controversial [87,88].

We have recently studied patients with COPD, evaluating lung parameters and antioxidant parameters, due to a possible involvement of OS in NTIS.

COPD is a complex condition, which cannot be considered a lung-related disorder, but rather a systemic disease also associated to increased oxidative stress. We evaluated thyroid hormones and antioxidant systems, the lipophilic CoQ_{10} and total antioxidant capacity (TAC) in COPD patients to reveal the presence of a low-T_3 syndrome in COPD and investigate the correlation between thyroid hormones, lung function parameters and antioxidants. The evaluation of CoQ_{10} was particularly interesting, also for the energetic role of this molecule, which is a component of the mitochondrial respiratory chain, as above stated; its concentrations were also corrected for cholesterol, due to its lipophilic nature. We studied 32 COPD patients and 45 controls; CoQ10 was assayed by HPLC; TAC by the metmyoglobin-ABTS method and expressed as latency time (LAG) in radical species appearance. We found significantly lower LAG values, fT_3 and fT_4 levels and significantly higher TSH in COPD patients vs controls. LAG values significantly correlated with fT_3 concentration. Twelve out of 32 patients exhibited fT_3 levels lower than normal range. When dividing COPD patients in two groups on the basis of the fT_3 concentration (normal fT_3 COPD and low fT_3 COPD), we observed lower LAG values in normal fT_3-COPD, compared to healthy subjects, with a further significant reduction in low fT_3-COPD patients. Moreover higher TSH concentration were present in normal fT_3-COPD, compared to healthy subjects, with a further significant increase in low fT_3-COPD patients. CoQ_{10}/cholesterol ratio was higher in low fT_3-COPD vs normal fT_3-COPD, with a nearly significant difference. These data seem to indicate an increased oxidative stress in low fT_3-COPD and a role of fT_3 in modulating antioxidant systems. However low fT_3 levels are joined to metabolic indexes of true hypothyroidism, suggesting that elevated CoQ_{10} expresses a reduced tissue utilization. Interestingly, there was no significant difference in lung parameters when comparing normal- or low-fT_3 COPD patients, according to the definition of COPD as a systemic disease, with respiratory parameters unable to define the severity of disease. In fact metabolic dysfunctions (i.e. osteoporosis, vascular and cardiac involvement, muscle impairment) play a role in the natural history of disease but were found poorly related to respiratory impairment, underlying the need of indexes related to a real tissue condition; the pattern of fT_3 could indicate such a situation, as reinforced by the pattern of CoQ_{10} levels; decreased plasma antioxidant capacity and increased CoQ_{10} levels in low fT_3-COPD, again suggested a possible condition of hypothyroidism at tissue levels [91].

The thyroid function has also been investigated in patients with acute kidney injury. It is known that TSH levels inversely correlated with urea concentrations and 82.9% of patients with kidney's disorders exhibited alteration in thyroid function, especially low-T_3. The thyroidal situation was ameliorated by improvement of renal function. No prognostic role was attributed to this dysfunction [92]. Primary hypothyroidism (non-autoimmune) is often observed in patients with chronic kidney disease (CKD); in particular the prevalence of subclinical hypothyroidism is related to GRF decline [93]. The earliest and the most common thyroid function abnormality in CKD patients is a low T_3 level (especially TT_3 than fT3) [94]. In the T_3 decreasing in this condition many mechanism are involved: fasting, chronic metabolic acidosis and chronic protein malnutrition, influencing T_4 deiodination, as well as protein binding of T_3. Besides the expression of type 1 5'- deiodinase, which is responsible for peripheral conversion of T_4 to T_3 [95], is inhibit by inflammatory cytokines such as tumor necrosis factor (TNF)-α and interleukin (IL)-1 causing a prolonged Wolff – Chaikoff effect [96]. In patients with CKD hormonal markers have a prognostic role: the low fT3 have been correlated with higher levels of markers of inflammation [highly sensitive C-reactive protein (hsCRP), IL-6, etc.], malnutrition (lower prealbumin, IGF-1), increased endothelial dysfunction, poorer cardiac function, poor survival, and higher all-cause as well as cardiovascular mortality in some studies [95, 97].

Even if there are TH alterations in acute liver failure (ALF), little is known about this topic [98]. An animal model was investigated (pigs subjected to surgical liver devascularisation). In this case serum T_4 and T_3 levels were markedly decreased, but fT_3 and TSH did not change. In the ALF there is a downregulation of T_4 and T_3 levels that seems to correlate with the severity if disease and was also related to alteration in parameters of inflammation, oxidative stress and myocardial thyroid receptors; thus the mechanisms in this case seem to be very complex. In humans acute liver failure (ALF) has hormonal implications, as has been recently shown for the hepatoadrenal syndrome [99], since an unexpected incidence of adrenal failure was discovered in ALF and post-transplantation patients; a glucocorticoid treatment can influence outcome. Also in chronic liver failure have been described thyroid function alterations [100-102], in particular has been described, in a subgroup of patients with cirrhosis at risk for decreased survival, a low T_4-variant of NTIS [100]; serum levels of fT_3 and TT_4 (but not TT_3 and fT_4) were significantly lower in patients with hepatic encephalopathy compared to decompensated cirrhotic patients without encephalopathy [102]. Much less clear data are available for ALF [103, 104]. In cirrhotic and also in acutely ill patients from various etiologies, derangements of thyroid hormones are common (up to 79% in the latter group, as reported from autoptic observations) [105].

Subclinical Hypothyroidism

Sublinical hypothyroidism (SH) is a condition characterized by slightly elevated TSH concentrations, in presence of normal TH levels. This is a biochemical definition, underlying that no overt clinical signs or symptoms are present [39]. It therefore denotes a balanced thyroid disfunction: it is debated if it represents an early stage of hypothyroidism which should be corrected by replacement therapy or not. The evolution of this condition is similarly uncertain.

Various clinical questions concern different aged population. A recent meta-analysis suggest that SH in children is a remitting process with low risk of evolution toward overt hypothyroidism [106]. The rate of evolution is between 0 and 28.8%; only one study report a percentage of 50% [107], but in a very small population. Risk factors are: elevated titer of thyroglobulin andibodies, presence of goiter, concomitance of celiac disease; dynamic evaluation during a long period of observation is however mandatory. Thyroxine treatment influences growth velocity and thyroid volume in such kind of subjects.

The same dilemma about the need of replacement therapy regards elderly population [108]. The prevalence of SH in older people is increasing and reported to be about 14% [109]. The hypothesis of increased risk for coronary heart disease and heart failure in SH is supported by two recent papers [110-111], suggesting a positive effect of treatment. This hypothesis was tested in a study, involving people with TSH levels in a range of 5-10 mUI/l, who received treatment and showed benefits, considering ischemic heart events and cardiovascular mortality [112]. In the same study, treatment was less effective in the older category (patients greater than 70 ys). To clarify this point a following study was performed in a very large population of non-institutionalized, categorized according to TSH levels. After adjusting the results for interferying variables (such as initiation of therapy, spontaneous fluctuations of TSH levels, the degree of SH, other cardiovascular risk factors), the authors did not find any increased risk for heart disease, heart failure or cardiovascular death in such patients. It can be hypothesized that TSH levels express a different meaning in older people, due to a reduced expression or activity of type 2 deiodinase, the main enzyme involved in the conversion from T_4 to T_3, again heading to the question of NTIS, especially when nutritional factors are present or other systemic disease influence thyroid hormone levels and metabolism, as above reported.

An important field is the effect on reproductive system [113]. Many studies have been performed also in subclinical hypothyroidism (SCH); the prevalence of SCH in infertile women was 11% in one study [114], but it is not considered as an infertility factors by others [115]. A positive correlation was found in early follicular phase between basal TSH, LH and T_4; moreover women with elevated TSH response to TRH had lower pregnancy rate than women with normal TSH response [116]. In a controlled prospective study of 438 women with infertility due to different causes, the median TSH levels were significantly higher than controls [117]. Moreover more frequent miscarriages were observed in women with higher basal TSH levels, irrespective of the presence of autoimmune thyroid disease (AITD) [118].

We want to focus our attention on luteal deficiency, on one side, and AITD, the most prevalent associated etiology in patients of reproductive age, on the other one. Progesterone secreted by the corpus luteum plays an important role in the maintenance of early pregnancy. Immediately after implantation, under the influence of human chorionic gonadotropin (hCG) secreted by the trophoblast, the corpus luteum receives a signal to continue in producing 17-α-progesterone together with estradiol, estrone, and relaxin [119-120]. The corpus luteum maintains its capacity to synthesize progesterone almost throughout the pregnancy, but at approximately 7 weeks gestation, its functional ability decreases markedly at the start of the luteoplacental transition. The removal of the corpus luteum before the eighth week of gestation results in abortion, whereas after the ninth week it does not [121]. Abnormalities of the luteal phase have been reported to occur in up to 35% of women with recurrent pregnancy losses [122]. There are several causes for determining luteal phase deficiency, including stress, exercise, weight loss, hyperprolactinemia, and menstrual cycles at the onset of puberty or perimenopause.

Luteal phase deficiency (LPD) may occur without any significant change in menstrual cycle lenght, despite prolonged follicular phases and shortened and/or progesterone-deficient secretion [123]. Clinically, LPD is associated with abnormal corpus luteal function, which includes the mentionated short luteal phases and inadequate progesterone production, and also inappropriate endometrial stimulation and maturation [124]. These luteal phase alterations cause asynchronous follicular growth, compromised oocyte maturation, and differentiated (out of phase) function of the endometrium, which is associated with low rates of cycle fecundity and high rates of embryonic loss, i.e. infertility and spontaneous abortion [124].

As above stated, hypoactive thyroid function is associated with infertility, even if severe forms of hypothyroidism rarely complicate pregnancy because they are associated with anovulation. However, in mild hypothyroidism, pregnancies can occur, but are associated with higher rates of pregnancy loss and maternal complications [125,126]. Even if an association exists between low thyroid function and pregnancy loss, a direct evidence for a causal role is missing [127]. One hypothesis for this correlation is that luteal phase defect has been linked to thyroid hypofunction. In consideration that production of progesterone is a pivotal element of a successful pregnancy, it is possible that pregnancy loss could be related to a deficient corpus luteum function [128].

An important study was published by Negro et al [129] showing, in a large cohort of women, that patients with positive thyroid autoantibodies (TPO-ab), even if euthyroid at the early stages of pregnancy, would benefit from L-thyroxine administration improving outcome of pregnancy, and namely reducing the rate of spontaneous miscarriage and premature delivery. Ab-positive pregnant women were significantly older than control population (suggesting that AITD could delay conception due to its relation with infertility) but exhibit a mean serum TSH, although normal, significantly higher than controls; women were randomized assigned to two groups, one without treatment, and the other with L-thyroxine treatment. In no-treated women, serum TSH progressively increased during gestation, in the meantime serum fT_4 decreased by 30%, suggesting reduced functional thyroid reserve due to AITD. On the contrary, in treated group, the miscarriage rate was reduced by 75% and frequency of premature delivery by 69%. Similar results were reported by other authors showing that age, TPO positivity and high TSH levels were independently associated with the risk of miscarriage in multivariate analysis [130]. An association between miscarriage and AITD had been previously described [131-132] and support in other population studies, confirming this association also in the case of apparent normal thyroid function [133]. A recent review separately considered association of AITD and miscarriage, AITD and recurrent miscarriage and finally AITD and early pregnancy loss after in vitro fertilization [134]. Finally another confirmation came from a meta-analysis of all case-controlled and longitudinal studies, with a 3-fold increased risk. Poppe et al. performed a prospective cohort study in women undergoing the first Assisted Reprudaction Technology (ART) cycle, excluding over thyroid dysfunction. The prevalence of antiTPO was 14%, without differences in TSH, fT_4 and age; in this ab-positive group, pregnancy rate was 53% vs 43%, with an odds ratio of 0.67, but in pregnant group the miscarriage rate was 53% and 23% respectively, with and odds ratio of 3.77 [135]. Autoimmune thyroiditis are clearly associated with clinically relevant events occurring before, during and after pregnancy [136]. Of course this strong association might be related to a generalized autoimmune disorders or a subtle thyroid hormone deficiency.

In this sense, a light is brought by studies performed with the administration of L-thyroxine. Vaquero et al [137] in patients with Ab positivity and two previous first-trimester miscarriage, treated with L-thyroxine, demonstred a better pregnancy outcome than untreated patients (81% vs 55%). Negro reported a reduction of miscarriage rate after L-thyroxine treatment in Ab positive infertile women who underwent in vitro fertilization [129]. Finally, Abalovich et al. [138] underlined the importance of adequate hormone treatment, comparing patients with hypothyroidism already known before pregnancy (adequate treatment) and patients with uncompletely adjusted replacement therapy: the pregnancy ended with abortion in 60% and 71% of cases, respectively.

In conclusion we believe it is prudent to screen for thyroid disease and normalize thyroid functions, when these are found abnormal, prior to conception above all if menstrual cycles are abnormal because of ovulation disturbance. Besides Ab+ women should be carefully evaluated before pregnancy for sublinical hypothyroidism.

We obtained personal data on subclinical hypothyroidism, in couples users of Billings Ovulation Method (BOM) for natural family planning; the Method is based on vulvar observation of the "Mucus Symptom", whose pattern is an accurate and precise marker of the ovarian function [139], validated by laboratory research and field trials [140, 141]. The BOM can be useful in studying clinical effects of subtle abnormalities in thyroid-gonadotropin interaction; the simple identification of the mucus peak as marker of ovulation and the evaluation of luteal phase length allow to detect a precise timing to perform hormonal assays. Therefore, we used the BOM to evaluate the prevalence of subclinical hypothyroidism in women, using the method for achieving or spacing pregnancy, with abnormal mucus pattern, not related to cervical pathology. Preliminary data were collected in 53 couples consulting our Center [142]; 22 of them exhibited an history of infertility (1-4 ys), with a range age of women: 26-42 ys. Evaluation of progesterone levels was performed on the 6th-7th day after the "peak of mucus symptom", or on the 6th-7th day before the expected menses, when no peak occurred. We evaluated basal plasma levels of fT_3, fT_4, TSH, PRL and performed a TRH test (200 ug iv, with TSH evaluation at 0, 30, 60 min) when TSH was normal or high normal. The presence of anti-TPO and anti-thyroglobulin autoantibodies was also evaluated. Subclinical hypothyroidism was defined as TSH peak response > 15 μg/ml, according to previous studies and comparison with age-matched controls [143].

Normal fT_3, fT_4 and PRL levels were present in all patients. Basal TSH was in high-normal range, with a TRH test diagnostic for subclinical hypothyroidism in 80% (n=42); prevalence of thyroid autoantibodies: 10%. Among the group of subclinical hypothyrodism, women were classified in three groups according to the BOM mucus symptom different patterns: anovulatory pattern of the mucus symptom (n=2), post-peak phases shortened and/or affected by spotting (n=22), normal lenght of luteal phase, but P in the lower range of postovulatory values (n=18); in the third group two women presented hypermenorrhea. Mean (±SEM) peak TSH response to TRH was 24.5 ± 1.5, 21.2 ± 1.5 and 22.5 ± 1.3 μU/ml, respectively.

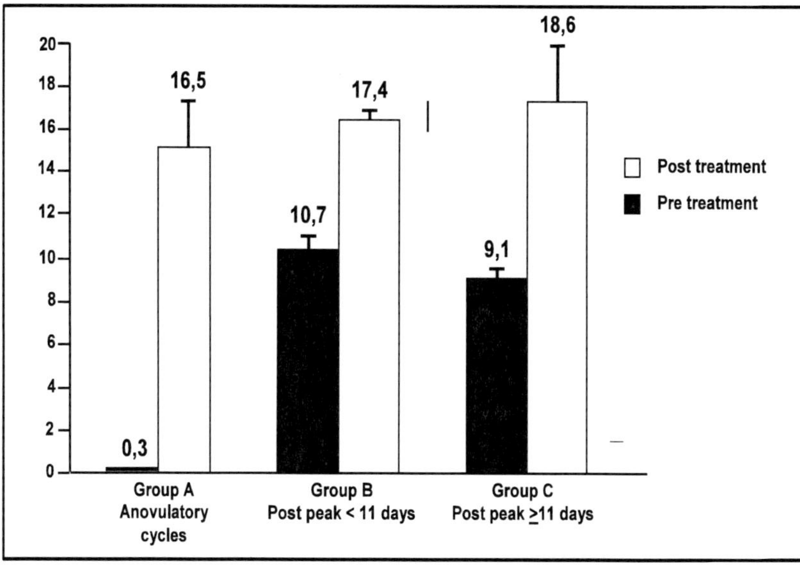

Figure 2. Post-peak (according to BOM) Progesterone levels (ng/ml) before and after replacement l-T4 treatment (from Mancini et al, Hypothyroidism, Oxidative stress and Reproduction, 2012, InTech Open book).

After L-thyroxine treatment, we observed a clear and significant increase in progesterone levels (evaluated 6-7 day after the “peak” of the “mucus symptom”), normal length of the post peak phase in all patients and the recovery of ovulation in the two women with anovulatory cycles (Fig. 2), strongly supporting a pathogenetic role of hypothyroidism in ovulation disturbances or luteal failure.

An hypothesis linking thyroid dysfunction and luteal deficiency is that concerning OS. Oxidative stress is associated with decreased female fertility in animals and in vitro models, but some observations in humans also reinforce this concept. Exposures associated with OS (extremes of body weight, alcohol, tobacco and caffeine intake) may induce pregnancy complications (e.g. preeclampsia); while intake of antioxidants nutrients, included use of multivitamins, have a beneficial role in female fertility [144]. More recently, it has been hypothesized that the exposure to environmental pollutants in fetal life may alter DNA methylation, causing altered gene expression in adult life [145, 146]; therefore this widespread condition should be added to the factors favouring OS. A role of reduced antioxidant defence has also been hypothesized in polycystic ovary, unexplained infertility and outcome of in vitro fertilization [147].

Conclusion

In summary, physiopathological studies suggest a condition of tissue hypothyroidism in both the two conditions analyzed in this report. This could be a rationale for treating these disorders; in the case of NTIS a vicious cyrcle can lead, despite its adaptive purpose, to a metabolic unfavourable condition for tissues such as brain and heart; in the case of subclinical hypothyroidism, this term often underestimates the clinical impact on symptoms such as ovarian function and risk of miscarriage. Probably, a full understanding of molecular mechanisms, which cause or are a consequence of low T_3 levels, will allow to choose patients who will really can have a benefit from replacement therapy and the appropriate schedule of treatment in NTIS. Subclinical hypothyroidism also should be considered a hypothyroid state, which should be differentiated by the lack of TSH suppression by reduced intrapituitary conversion from T_4 to T_3.

References

[1] Zhu, X; Cheng, S.Y. New insights into regulation of lipid metabolism by thyroid hormone. *Curr Opin Endocrinol Diab Obes*, 2010, 17, 408-413.

[2] Crane, FL. Biochemical functions of coenzyme Q10. *J Am Coll Nutr,* 2001, 20(6), 591-598.

[3] Kostic, I; Curcio, F. Causes of Hypothyroidism. In: Drahomira Springer, Editor. *Hypothyroidism – Influences and Treatments*. Rijeka: InTech; 2012; pp. 161-172.

[4] Hollowell, JG; Staehling, NW; Flanders, WD; Hannon, WH; Gunter, EW; Spencer, CA; Braverman, LE. Serum TSH, T(4), and thyroid antibodies in the United States population (1988 to 1994): National Health and Nutrition Examination Survey (NHANES III*). J Clin Endocrinol Metab*, 2002, 87(2), 489–499.

[5] Vanderpump, MP; Tunbridge, WM; French, JM, Appleton, D; Bates, D; Clark, F; Grimley Evans, J; Hasan, DM; Rodgers, H; Tunbridge, F; et al. The incidence of thyroid disorders in the community: a twenty-year follow-up of the Whickham Survey. *Clin Endocrinol* (Oxf). 1995; 43(1), 55–68.

[6] Leese, GP; Flynn, RV; Jung, RT; Macdonald, TM; Murphy, MJ; Morris, AD. Increasing prevalence and incidence of thyroid disease in Tayside, Scotland: the Thyroid Epidemiology Audit and Research Study (TEARS). *Clin Endocrinol*, 2008, 68(2), 311–316.

[7] Tunbridge, WM; Evered, DC; Hall, R; Appleton, D; Brewis, M; Clark, F; Evans, JG; Young, E; Bird, T; Smith, PA. The spectrum of thyroid disease in a community: the Whickham survey. *Clin Endocrinol*, 1977, 7(6), 481–493.

[8] Van den Beld, AW; Visser, TJ; Feelders, RA; Grobbee, DE; Lamberts, SW. Thyroid hormone concentrations, disease, physical function, and mortality in elderly men. *J Clin Endocrinol Metab*, 2005, 90(12), 6403–6409.

[9] Chakera, AJ; Pearce, SH; Vaidya, B. Treatment for primary hypothyroidism: current approaches and future possibilities. *Drug Des Devel Ther*, 2012, 6, 1-11.

[10] Rastogi, MV; LaFranchi, SH. Congenital hypothyroidism. *Orphanet J Rare Dis,* 2010, 10, 5-17.

[11] Brent, GA; Davies TF. Hypothyroidism and thyroiditis. In: Melmed, S; Polonsky, KS; Reed Larsen, P; Kronenberg HM, Editors. Williams

Textbook of Endocrinology, 12 th Ed, Philadelphia, Elsevier Saunders; 2011; pp. 406-439.

[12] Tulloch, B.R. Lipid Changes in Thyroid Disease: The Effect of Thyroxine and Analogues. *Proceeding of the Royal Society of Medicine*, Vol.67, No.7; 1974; pp. 670-671.

[13] Choi, JW; Choi, HS. The regulatory effects of thyroid hormone on the activity of 3-hydroxy-3-methylglutaryl coenzyme A reductase. *Endocr Res,* 2000, 26, 1–21.

[14] Tzotzas, T; Krassas, GE; Konstantinidis, T; Bougoulia, M. Changes in lipoprotein(a) levels in overt and subclinical hypothyroidism before and during treatment. *Thyroid*, 2000, 10(9), 803-808.

[15] Erqou, S.; Kaptoge, S.; Perry, PL; Di Angelantonio, E; Thompson, A; White, IR; Marcovina, SM; Collins, R; Thompson, SG; Danesh, J Lipoprotein(a) concentration and the risk of coronary heart disease, stroke, and nonvascular mortality. *JAMA*, 2009, 302(4), 412-423.

[16] Pearce, EN. Update in Lipid Alterations in Subclinical Hypothyroidism. *J Clin Endocrinol Metab*, 2012, 97, 326 –333.

[17] Dullaart, RP; Hoogenberg, K; Groener, JE; Dikkeschei, LD; Erkelens, DW, Doorenbos, H. The activity of cholesteryl ester transfer protein is decreased in hypothyroidism: a possible contribution to alterations in high-density lipoproteins. *Eur J Clin Invest*, 1990, 20(6) 581-587.

[18] De Groot, L. "Non-thyroidal illness syndrome" is a manifestation of hypothalamic-pituitary dysfunction, and in the view of current evidence, should be treated with appropriate replacement therapies. *Crit Care Clin,* 2006, 22(1), 57-86.

[19] Mancini, A; Raimondo, S; Di Segni, C; Persano, M; Pontecorvi, A. Non-Thyroidal Illness: Physiopathology and Clinical Implications. In: Potluková, E. *Current Topics in Hypothyroidism with Focus on Development*, Rijeka: InTech; 2013; pp. 183-202.

[20] Rubenfeld, S. Euthyroid sick syndrome. *N Engl J Med,* 1978, 299(25), 1414-1415.

[21] Wartofsky, L; Burman, KD. Alterations in thyroid function in patients with systemic illness: the "Euthyroid sick syndrome*". Endocr Rev*, 1982, 3, 164-217.

[22] Chopra IJ. Euthyroid sick syndrome: abnormalities in circulating thyroid hormones and thyroid hormone physiology in illness (NTI). *Med Grand Rounds* 1982;1 201–212.

[23] Chopra, IJ; Chopra, U; Smith, SR; Reza, M; Solomon, DH. Reciprocal changes in serum concentrations of 3,3',5-triiodothyronine (T3) in systemic illnesses. *J Clin Endocrinol Metab*, 1975, 41, 1043–1049.
[24] Umpierrez, GE. Euthyroid Sick Syndrome. *South Med J*, 2002, 95(5), 506-513.
[25] Michalaki, M; Vagenakis, AG; Makri, M; Kalfarentzos, F; Kyriazopoulou, V. Dissociation of the early decline in serum T(3)concentration and serum IL-6 rise and TNF-alpha in illness syndrome induced by abdominal surgery. *J Clin Endocrinol Metab*, 2001, 86, 4198– 4205.
[26] Chopra, IJ. Clinical review 86: Euthyroid sick syndrome: is it a misnomer? *J Clin Endocrinol Metab*, 1997, 82, 329–334.
[27] Bermudez, F; Surks, MI; Oppenheimer, JH. High incidence of decreased serum triiodothyronine concentration in patients with non thyroidal disease. *J Clin Endocrinol Metab*, 1975, 41, 27–40.
[28] Kaplan, MM; Larsen, PR; Crantz, FR; Dzau, VJ; Rossing, TH; Haddow, JE. Prevalence of abnormal thyroid function test results in patients with acute medical illnesses. *Am J Med*, 1982, 72 9–16.
[29] Marx, C; Petros, S; Bornstein, SR; Weise, M; Wendt, M; Menschikowski, M; Engelmann, L; Hoffken, G. Adrenocortical hormones in survivors and nonsurvivors of severe sepsis: diverse time course of dehydroepiandrosterone, dehydroepiandrosterone-sulfate, and cortisol. *Crit Care Med* 2003, 31, 1382–1388.
[30] Schuetz, P; Muller, B; Nusbaumer, C; Wieland, M; Christ-Crain, M. Circulating levels of GH predict mortality and complement prognostic scores in critically ill medical patients. *Eur J Endocrinol,* 2009, 160, 157-163.
[31] Van den Berghe, G; De Zegher, F; Bouillon, R. Acute and prolonged critical illness as different neuroendocrine paradigms. *J Clin Endocrinol Metab,* 1998, 83, 1827-1834.
[32] Van den Berghe, G. Dynamic neuroendocrine responses to critical illness. *Frontiers Neuroendocrinol*, 2002, 23, 370-391.
[33] Mancini, A; Corbo, GM; Gaballo, A; Valente, S; Gigliotti, P; Cimino, V; De Marinis, L; Principi, F; Littarru, GP. Relationships between plasma CoQ10 levels and thyroid hormones in chronic obstructive pulmonary disease. *Biofactors*, 2005, 25 (1-4), 201-204.
[34] Peeters, RP; Wouters, PJ; Kaptein, E; van Toor, H; Visser, TJ; Van den Berghe, G. Reduced activation and increased inactivation of thyroid

hormone in tissues of critically ill patients. *J Clin Endocrinol Metab*, 2003, 88 (7), 3202-3211.

[35] Luca, F; Goichot, B; Brue, T. Non thyroidal illnesses (NTIS). *Ann Endocrinol* (Paris), 2010, 71 (Suppl 1) S 13- 24.

[36] Economidou, F; Douka, E; Tzanela, M; Nanas, S; Kotanidou, A. Thyroid function during critical illness. *Hormones*, 2011, 10 (2), 117-124.

[37] Bello, G; Ceaichisciuc, I; Silva, S; Antonelli, M. The role of thyroid dysfunction in the critically ill: a review of literature. *Minerva Anestesiol,* 2010, 76 (11), 919-928.

[38] Magagnin Wajner, S; Maia, AL. New insights toward the acute non thyroidal illness syndrome. *Front Endocrinol*, 2012, 3 (8) 1-7.

[39] Biondi, B. Natural history, diagnosis and management of subclinical thyroid dysfunction; *Best Pract Res Clin Endocrinol Metab*, 2012, 26, 431–446.

[40] Brent, GA; Hershman, JM; Reed, AW; Sastre, A; Lieberman, J. Serum angiotensin converting enzyme in severe nonthyroidal illness associated with low serum thyroxine concentration. *Ann Intern Med*, 1986, 100:680- 683.

[41] Krassas, GE; Poppe, K; Glinoer, D. Thyroid function and human reproductive health. *Endocr Rev,* 2010, 31(5), 702-55.

[42] Ruder, H; Corvol, P; Mahoudeau, JA; Ross, GT; Lipsett, MB. Effects of induced hyperthyroidism on steroid me- tabolism in man. *J Clin Endocrinol Metab,* 1971, 33, 382–387.

[43] Vermeulen, A; Verdonck, L; Van der Straeten, M; Orie, N. Capacity of the testosterone-binding globulin in human plasma and influence of specific binding of testosterone on its metabolic clearance rate. *J Clin Endocrinol Metab,* 1969, 29, 1470–1480.

[44] Donnelly, P; White, C. Testicular dysfunction in men with primary hypothyroidism; reversal of hypogonadotro-phic hypogonadism with replacement thyroxine. *Clin Endocrinol* (Oxf), 2000, 52, 197–201.

[45] Cavaliere, H; Abelin, N; Medeiros-Neto, G Serum levels of total testosterone and sex hormone binding globulin in hypothyroid patients and normal subjects treated with incremental doses of L-T4 or L-T3. *J Androl,* 1988, 9, 215–219.

[46] Salerno, M; Micillo, M; Di Maio, S; Capalbo, D; Ferri, P; Lettiero, T; Tenore, A Longitudinal growth, sexual maturation and final height in patients with congenital hypothyroidism detected by neonatal screening. *Eur J Endocrinol,* 2001, 145:377–383.

[47] Meikle, AW. The interrelationships between thyroid dysfunction and hypogonadism in men and boys. *Thyroid*, 2004, 14 (Suppl 1), S17–S25.
[48] Kocova, M; Netkov, S; Sukarova-Angelovska, E. Pitu- itary pseudotumor with unusual presentation reversed shortly after the introduction of thyroxine replacement therapy. *J Pediatr Endocrinol Metab* 2001, 14, 1665–1669
[49] Horvath, E; Kovacs, K; Scheithauer, BW. *Pituitary hyperplasia. Pituitary*, 1999, 1, 169 –179.
[50] Seppel, T; Becker, A; Lippert, F; Schlaghecke, R. Serum sex hormone-binding globulin and osteocalcin in systemic nonthyroidal illness associated with low thyroid hormone concentrations. *J Clin Endocrinol Metab*, 1996, 81, 1663-1665.
[51] Wenzel, KW. Recent parameters for diagnosis of challenging thyroid gland disorders: consequences for diagnosis and therapy. *Acta Med Austriaca*, 1991, 18(1), 1-6.
[52] Mundy, GR. Regulation of bone formation by bone morphogenetic proteins and other growth factors. *Clin Orthop Relat Res*, 1996, 324, 24-28.
[53] Littarru, GP; Tiano L. Clinical aspects of Coenzyme Q10: an update. *Nutrition*, 2010, 26(3), 250-254.
[54] Kaltschmidt, B; Sparna, T; Kaltschmidt, C. Activation of NF-kappa B by reactive oxygen intermediates in the nervous system. *Antioxid Redox Signal,* 1999, 1, 129-44.
[55] Mosca, F; Fattorini, D; Bompadre, S; Littarru, GP. Assay of coenzymeQ10 in plasma by a single dilution step. *Anal Biochem*, 2002, 305, 49-54.
[56] Littarru, GP; Tiano, L. Clinical aspects of coenzyme Q10: an update. *Curr Opin Clin Nutr Metab Care*, 2005, 8, 641-646.
[57] Mancini, A; De Marinis, L; Calabrò, F; Sciuto, R; Oradei, A; Lippa, S; Sandric, S; Litarru, GP; Barbarino A. Evaluation of metabolic status in amiodarone-induced thyroid disorders: plasma coenzyme Q10 determination. *J. Endocrinol Invest*, 1989, 12, 511-516.
[58] Bianchi, G; Solaroli, E; Zaccheroni, V; Grossi, G; Bargossi, AM; Melchionda, M; Marchesini, G. Oxidative stress and antioxidant metabolites in patients with hyperthyroidism: effect of treatment. *Horm Metab Res,* 1999, 31, 620-624.
[59] Mancini, A; Conte, G; De Marinis, L; Oradei, A; Littarru, GP. Thyroid hormone and oxidative metabolism: Coenzyme Q10 in thyroid's disease. *CoQ Biol Med*, 1993, 1, 25-34.

[60] Roncoroni, R; Beck-Peccoz, P; Fornasini, GF; Preziati, D; Paccagnini, O; Persani, L; Carenzi, A; Faglia, G. Il dosaggio dei livelli circolanti di ubidecarenone (CoQ10) quale parametro di valutazione dell'azione periferica degli ormoni tiroidei. *Abstracts of the 7th "Giornate Italiane della Tiroide"*, S. Margherita Ligure, 1989, p. 67 (abstract).
[61] Mancini, A; Corbo, GM; Gaballo, A; Valente, S; Cimino V; Gigliotti, P; DE Marinis L; Principi, F; Littarru, GP. Relationships between CoQ10 levels and thyroid hormones in chronic obstructive pulmonary disease. *Abstracts of the 4th Conference of the International Coenzyme Q10 Association*, Los Angeles, 14-17 aprile 2005, p. 146
[62] Lewis, SE; Boyle, PM; McKinney, KA; Young, IS; Thompson, W. Total antioxidant capacity of seminal plasma is different in fertile and infertile men. *Fertil Steril*, 1995, 64, 868-8770.
[63] Rice-Evans, C; Miller, NJ. Total antioxidant status in plasma and body fluids. *Methods Enzymol*, 1994, 234, 279-293.
[64] Meucci, E; Milardi, D; Mordente, A; Martorana, GE; Giacchi, E; De Marinis, L; Mancini A. Total antioxidant capacity in patients with varicoceles. *Fertil Steril*, 2003, 79 (Suppl 3), 1577-1583.
[65] Mancini, A; Festa, R; Di Donna, V; Leone, E; Littarru, GP; Silvestrini, A; Meucci, E; Pontecorvi A. Hormones and antioxidant systems: Role of pituitary and pituitary-dependent axes. *J Endocrinol Invest*, 2010, 33, 422-433.
[66] Mancini, A; Leone, E; Silvestrini, A; Festa, R; Di Donna, V; De Marinis, L; Pontecorvi, A; Littarru, GP; Meucci, E. Evaluation of antioxidant systems in pituitary-adrenal axis diseases. *Pituitary*, 2010, 13, 138-145.
[67] Mancini, A; Leone, E; Festa, R; Grande, G; De Marinis, L; Pontecorvi, A; Maira, G; Littarru, GP; Meucci, E. Effects of testosterone on antioxidant systems in male secondary hypogonadism. *J Androl*, 2008, 29, 622-629.
[68] Henneman, G; Docter, R; Krenning, EP. Causes and effects of the low T3 syndrome during caloric deprivation and non-thyroidal illness: an overview. *Acta Med Austriaca*, 1988, 15 42-45.
[69] Monig, H; Arendt, T; Meyer, M; Kloehn, S; Bewig, B. Activation of the hypothalamo- pituitary-adrenal axis in response to septic or non-septic diseases- implications for the euthyroid sick syndrome. *Intensive Care Med,* 1999, 25, 1402-1406.

[70] Cherem, HJ; Nellen, HH; Barabejski, FG; Chong, MBA; Lifshits, GA. Thyroid function and abdominal surgery. A longitudinal study. *Arch Med Res*, 1992, 23 143-147.

[71] Ilias, I; Stamoulis, K; Armaganidis, A; Lyberopoulos, P; Tzanela, M; Orfanos, S; Theodorakopoulou, M; Tsagarakis, S; Dimopoulou, I. Contribution of endocrine parameters in predicting outcome of multiple trauma patients in an intensive care unit. *Hormones*, 2007, 6 218-226.

[72] Vardarli, I; Schmidt, R; Wdowinski, JM; Teuber, J; Schwedes, U; Usadel, KH. *The hypo- thalamo-hypophyseal thyroid axis, plasma protein concentration and the hypophy- seogonadal axis in low T3 syndrome following acute myocardial infarct.* Klinische Wochenschrift 1987, 65, 129-133.

[73] Hamilton, MA; Stevenson, LW; Lun, M; Walden, JA. Altered thyroid hormone metabolism in advanced heart failure. *J Am Coll Cardiol*, 1990, 16 (1), 91-95.

[74] Holland, FW; Brown, PS; Weintraub, BD; Clark, RE. Cardiopulmonary bypass and thyroid function: an "euthyroid sick syndrome". *Ann Thorac Surg*, 1991, 52, 46-50.

[75] Scoscia, E; Baglioni, S; Eslami, A; Iervasi, G; Monti, S; Todisco, T. Clinical study "Low triiodothyronine (T3) state: a predictor of outcome in respiratory failure? Results of a clinical pilot study. *Eur J Endocrinol*, 2004, 151, 557-560.

[76] Vexiau, P; Perez-Castiglioni P; Socie, G; Devergie, A; Toubert, ME; Aractingi, S; Gluckmann, E. The " Euthyroid sick syndrome": incidence, risk factors and prognostic value soon after allogenic bone marrow transplantation. *Br J Hematol*, 1993, 85, 778-782.

[77] Kaptein, EM. Clinical relevance of thyroid hormone alterations in non-thyroidal illness. *Thyroid International*, 1997, 4, 22-25.

[78] Wang, F; Pan, W; Wang, H; Wang, S; Pan, S; Ge, J. Relationship between thyroid function and ICU mortality: a prospective observation study. *Crit Care,* 2012, 16 (1), R11.

[79] Bello, G; Pennisi, MA; Montini, L; Silva, S; Maviglia, R; Cavallaro, F; Bianchi, A; De Marinis, L; Antonelli, M. Nonthyroidal illness syndrome and prolonged mechanical ventilation in patients admitted to the ICU. *Chest*, 2009, 135 (6), 1448-1454.

[80] Klein, I; Ojamaa, K. Thyroid hormone and the cardiovascular system. *N Engl J Med*, 2001, 344, 501-509.

[81] Franklyn, JA; Gammage, MD; Ramsden, DB; Sheppard, MC. Thyroid status in patients after acute myocardial infarction. *Clin Sci* (Lond), 1984, 67, 585-590.

[82] De Marinis, L; Mancini, A; Masala, R; Torlontano, M; Sandric, S; Barbarino, A. Evaluation of pituitary-thyroid axis response to acute myocardial infarction. *J Endocrinol Invest*, 1985, 8, 507-511.

[83] Chow, CC; Mak, TW; Chan, CH; Cockram, CS. Euthyroid sick syndrome in pulmonary tuberculosis before and after treatment. *Ann Clin Biochem*, 1995, 32, 385-391.

[84] Kawakami, M; Usami, I; Kuroki, H; Goto, M. *Thyroid hormones in patients with clinical stable pneumoconiosis*. Nihon Kyobu Shikkan Gakkai Zasshi, 1993, 31, 1215-1219.

[85] Wawrzynska, L; Sakowicz, A; Filipecki, S. Euthyroid sick syndrome in patients with respiratory failure. *Pneumol Alergol Pol*, 1996, 64 (Suppl 2), 193-199.

[86] Laghi, F; Adiguzel, N; Tobin, MJ. Endocrinological derangements in COPD. *Eur Respir J,* 2009, 34, 975-996.

[87] Dimopolou, I; Ilias, I; Mastorakos, G; Mantzos, E; Roussos, C; Koutras, DA. Effects of severity of chronic obstructive pulmonary disease on thyroid function. *Metabolism Clin Exper*, 2001, 50, 1397-1401.

[88] Okutan, O; Kartaloglu, Z; Onde, ME; Bozkanat, E; Kunter, E. Pulmonary function tests and thyroid hormone concentrations in patients with chronic obstructive pulmonary disease. *Med Princ Pract*, 2004, 13, 126-128.

[89] Karadag, F; Ozcan, H; Karul, AB; Yilmaz, M; Cildag, O. Correlates of non-thyroidal illness syndrome in chronic obstructive pulmonary disease. *Respir Med,* 2007, 101, 1439-1446.

[90] Bratel, T; Wennlund, A; Carlstrom, K. Impact of hypoxaemia on neuroendocrine function and catecholamine secretion in chronic obstructive pulmonary disease (COPD): Effects of long-term oxygen treatment. *Respir Med*, 2000, 94, 1221-1228.

[91] Mancini, A; Corbo, GM; Gaballo, A; Raimondo, S; Di Segni, C; Gigliotti, P; Silvestrini, A; Valente, S; Littarru, GP; Pontecorvi, A; Meucci E. Relationship between plasma antioxidants and thyroid hormones in chronic obstructive pulmonary disease. *Exp Clin Endocrinol Diab*, 2012, 120, 623-628.

[92] Iglesias, P; Olea, T; Vega-Cabrera, C; Heras, M; Bajo, MA; Del Peso, G; Arias, MJ; Selgas, R; Díez, JJ. Thyroid function tests in acute kidney injury. *J Nephrol,* 2013, 26(1), 164-172.

[93] Lo, JC; Chertow, GM; Go, AS; Hsu, CY. Increased prevalence of subclinical and clinical hypothyroidism in persons with chronic kidney disease. *Kidney Int*, 2005, 67, 1047-1052.
[94] Wiederkehr, MR; Kalogiros, J; Krapf, R. Correction of metabolic acidosis improves thyroid and growth hormone axes in haemodialysis patients. *Nephrol Dial Transplant*, 2004, 19, 1190-1197.
[95] Zoccali, C; Tripepi, G; Cutrupi, S; Pizzini, P; Mallamaci, F. Low triiodothyronine: A new facet of inflammation in end-stage renal disease. *J Am Soc Nephrol*, 2005, 16, 2789-2795.
[96] Bando, Y; Ushiogi, Y; Okafuji, K; Toya, D; Tanaka, N; Miura, S. Non-autoimmune primary hypothyroidism in diabetic and non-diabetic chronic renal dysfunction. *Exp Clin Endocrinol Diabetes*, 2002, 110, 408-415.
[97] Carrero, JJ; Qureshi, AR; Axelsson, J; Yilmaz, MI; Rehnmark, S; Witt, MR; Barany, P; Heimburger, O; Suliman, ME; Alvestand, A; Lindholm, B; Stenvinkel, P. Clinical and biochemical implications of low thyroid hormone levels (total and free forms) in euthyroid patients with chronic kidney disease. *J Intern Med,* 2007, 262, 690-701.
[98] Kostopanagiotou, G; Kalimeris, K; Mourouzis, I; Costopanagiotou, C; Arkadopoulos, N; Panagopoulos, D; Papoutsidakis, N; Chranioti, A; Pafiti, A; Spanou, D; Smyrniotis, V; Pantos, C. Thyroid hormones alterations during acute liver failure: possible underlying mechanisms and consequences. *Endocrine*, 2009, 36 (2), 198-204.
[99] Marik, PE; Gayowski, T; Starzl, TE. The hepatoadrenal syndrome: a common yet unrecognized clinical condition. *Crit Care Med*, 2005, 33, 1254-1259.
[100] Caregaro, L; Alberino, F; Amodio, P; Merkel, C; Angeli, P; Plebani, M; Gatta, A. Nutritional and prognostic significance of serum hypothyroxinemia in hospitalized patients with liver cirrhosis. *J Hepatol,* 1998, 28, 115-121.
[101] Zietz, B; Lock, G; Plach, B; Drobnik, W; Grossmann, J; Scholmercih, J; Straub, RH. Dys- function of the hypothalamic-pituitary-glandular axes and relation to Child-Pugh classification in male patients with alcoholic and virus-related cirrhosis. *Eur J Gastroenterol Hepatol*, 2003, 15, 495-501.
[102] Kayacetin, E; Kisakol, G; Kaya, A. Low serum total thyroxine and free triiodothyronine in patients with hepatic encephalopathy due to non-alcoholic cirrhosis. *Swiss Med Wkly*, 2003, 133, 210-213.

[103] Bratusch-Marrain, P; Vierhapper, H; Grubeck-Loebenstein, B; Waldhausl, W; Kleinberger, G. Pituitary-thyroid dysfunction in severe non-thyroidal disease: "low-T4 syndrome". *Endokrinologie*, 1982, 80, 207-212.

[104] Kaptein, EM; Robinson, WJ; Grieb, DA. Peripheral serum thyroxine, triiodothyronine and reverse triiodothyronine kinetics in the low state of acute nonthyroidal illnesses. *J Clin Invest,* 1982, 69, 526-535.

[105] Arem, R; Wiener, GJ; Kaplan, SG; Kim, HS; Reichlin, S; Kaplan, MM. Reduced tissue thyroid hormone levels in fatal illness. *Metabolism*, 1993, 42, 1102-1108.

[106] Monzani, A; Prodam, F; Rapa, A; Moia, S; Agarla, V; Bellone, S; Bona, G. Natural history of subclinical hypothyroidism in children and adolescents and potential effects of replacement therapy: a review. *Eur J Endocrinol,* 2013, 168, R1–R11.

[107] Jaruratanasirikul, S; Leethanaporn, K; Khuntigij, P; Sriplung, H. The clinical course of Hashimoto's thryoiditis in children and adolescents: 6 years longitudinal follow-up. *J Pediatr Endocrinol Metab*, 2001, 14, 177–184.

[108] Klein, I. Subclinical Hypothyroidism—Just a High Serum Thyrotropin (TSH) Concentration or Something Else? *J Clin Endocrinol Metab*, 2013, 98(2), 508–510.

[109] Hyland, KA; Arnold, AM; Lee, JS; Cappola, AR. Persistent subclinical hypothyroidism and cardiovascular risk in the elderly: the Cardiovascular Health Study. *J Clin Endocrinol Metab*, 2013, 98, 533–540.

[110] Rotondi, M; Magri, F; Chiovato, L. Risk of coronary heart disease and mortality for adults with subclinical hypothyroidism. *JAMA*, 2010, 304(22), 2481.

[111] Gencer, B; Collet, TH; Virgini, V; Bauer, DC; Gussekloo, J; Cappola, AR; Nanchen, D; den Elzen, WP; Balmer, P; Luben, RN; Iacoviello, M; Triggiani, V; Cornuz, J; Newman, AB; Khaw, KT; Jukema, JW; Westendorp, RG; Vittinghoff, E; Aujesky, D; Rodondi, N. Subclinical thyroid dysfunction and the risk of heart failure events: an individual participant data analysis from 6 prospective cohorts. *Circulation*, 2012, 126, 1040-1049.

[112] Razvi, S; Weaver, JU; Butler, TJ; Pearce, SH. Levothyroxine treatment of subclinical hypothyroidism, fatal and nonfatal cardiovascular events, and mortality. *Arch Intern Med*, 2012, 172, 811– 817.

[113] Mancini, A; Giacchi, E; Raimondo, S; Di Segni, C; Silvestrini, A, Meucci E. Hypothyroidism, Oxidative Stress and Reproduction. In:

Drahomira Springer, Editor. *Hypothyroidism – Influences and Treatments.* Rijeka: InTech; 2012; pp. 117-134.

[114] Bohnet, HG; Fielder, K; Leidenberger, FA. Subclinical hypothyroidism and infertility. *Lancet*, 1981, 2, 1278-1279.

[115] Bals-Pratsch, M; De Geyter, C; Muller, T; Frieling, U; Lerchl, A; Pirke, KM; Hanker, JP; Becker-Carus, C; Nieschlag, E. Episodic variations of prolactin, thyroid- stimulating hormone, luteinizing hormone, melatonin and cortisol in infertile women with sublinical hypothyroidism. *Hum Reprod,* 1997, 12, 896-904.

[116] Gerhard, I; Becker, T; Eggert-Kruse, W; Klinga, K; Runnebaum, B. Thyroid and ovarian function in infertile women. *Hum Reprod*, 1991, 6, 338-345.

[117] Poppe, K; Glinoer, D; Van Steirteghem, A; Tournaye, H; Devroey, P; Schiettecatte, J; Velkeniers, B. Thyroid dysfunction and autoimmunity in infertile women. *Thyroid*, 2002, 12, 997-1001.

[118] Raber, W; Nowotny, P; Vytiska-Binstorfer, E; Vierhapper, H. Thyroxine treatment modified in infertile women according to thyroxine-relasing hormone testing: 5 year follow-up of 283 women referred after exclusion of absolute causes of infertility. *Hum Reprod*, 2003, 18, 707-714.

[119] Szlachter, N; O'Byrne, E; Goldsmith, L; Steinetz, BG; Weiss G. Myometrial inhibiting activity of relaxin-containg extracts of human corpora lutea of pregnancy. Am J Obstet Gynecol, 1980, 136 (5), 584-586.

[120] Bigazzi, M; Nardi, E. Prolactin and relaxin: antagonism on the spontaneous motility of the uterus. *J Clin Endocrinol Metabol*, 1981, 53 (6), 665- 667.

[121] Csapo, AI; Pulkkinen, MO; Wiest, WG. Effects of luteectomy and progesterone replacement therapy in early pregnant patients. *Am J Obstet Gynecol*, 1973, 115 (6), 759-765.

[122] Insler, V. Corpus luteum defects. *Curr Opin Obstet Gynecol*, 1992, 4 (2), 203-211.

[123] De Souza, MJ; Miller, BE; Loucks, AB; Luciano, AA; Pescatello, LS; Campbell, CG; Lasley, BL. High frequency of luteal phase deficiency and anovulation in recreational women runners; blunted elevation in follicle-stimulating hormone observed during luteal-follicular transition. *J Clin Endocrinol Metab*, 1998, 83 (12), 4220-4232.

[124] Ginsburg, KA. Luteal phase defect. Etiology, diagnosis and management. *Endocrinol Metab Clin North Am*, 1992, 21 (1), 85-104.

[125] Davis, LE; Leveno, KJ; Cunningham, FG. Hypothyroidism complicating pregnancy. *Obstet Gynec*, 1988, 72 (1), 108-112.

[126] Stray-Pedersen, B; Tray-Pedersen, S. Etiologic factors and subsequent reproductive performances in 195 couples with a prior history of habitual abortion. *Am J Obstet Gynecol*, 1984, 148 (2),140-146.

[127] Clifford, K; Rai, R; Watson, H; Regan, L. An informative protocol for the investigation of recurrent miscarriage: preliminary experience of 5000 consecutive cases. *Hum Reprod*, 1994, 9 (7), 1328-1332.

[128] Daya, S; Ward, S; Burrows, E. Progesterone profiles in luteal phase defect cycles and outcome of progesterone treatment in patients with recurrent spontaneous abortion. *Am J Obstet Gynecol*, 1988, 158 (2), 225-232.

[129] Negro, R; Formoso, G; Mangieri, T; Pezzarossa, A; Dazzi, D; Hassan, H. Levothyroxine treatment in euthyroid pregnant women with autoimmune thyroid disease: effect on obstetrical complications. *J Clin Endocrinol Metabol,* 2006, 91, 2587-2591.

[130] Sieiro Netto, L; Medina Coeli, C; Micmacher, E; Ma mede Da Costa, S; Nazar, L; Galvao, D; Buescu, A; Vaisman, M. Influence of thyroid autoimmunity and maternal age on the risk of miscarriage. *Am J Reprod Immunol*, 2004, 52 (5), 312-316.

[131] Stagnaro-Green, A; Roman, SH; Cobin, RH; El-Hazary, E; Alvarez-Marfany, M; Davies, TF. Detection of at-risk pregnancy by means of highly sensitive assays for thyroid antibodies. *JAMA*, 1990, 264, 1422-1425.

[132] Glinoer, D; Fernandez Soto, ML; Bourdoux, P; Lejeune, B; Delange, F; Lemone, M; Klitheart, J; Robijn, C; Grun, JP; De Nayer, P. Pregnancy in patients with mild thyroid abnormalities: maternal and neonatal repercussions. *J Clin Endocrinol Metab*, 1991, 73, 421-427.

[133] Poppe, K; Glinoer, D. Thyroid autoimmunity and hypothyroidism before and during pregnancy. *Hum Reprod Update*, 2003, 9, 149-161.

[134] Stagnaro-Green, A; Glinoer, D. Thyroid autoimmunity and hypothyroidism before and during pregnancy. *Hum Reprod Update*, 2004, 9, 149-161.

[135] Poppe, K; Glinoer, D; Tournaye, H; Devroey, P; van Steirteghem, A; Kaufman, L; Velkeniers, B. Assisted reproduction and thyroid autoimmunity: an unfortunate combination? *J Clin Endocrinol Metab,* 2003, 88 (9), 4149-4152.

[136] Muller, AF; Berghout, A. Consequences of autoimmune thyroiditis before, during and after pregnancy. *Min Endocrinol*, 2003, 28 (3), 247-254.

[137] Vaquero, E; Lazzarin, N; De Carolis, C; Valensise, H; Moretti, C; Romanini, C. Mild thyroid abnormalities and recurrent spontaneous abortion: diagnostic and therapeutic approach. *Am J Reprod Immunol*, 2000, 43 (4), 204-208.

[138] Abalovich, M; Gutierrez, S; Alcaraz, G; Maccallini, G; Garcia, A; Levalle, O. Overt and subclinical hypothyroidism complicating pregnancy. *Thyroid*, 2002, 12, 63- 68.

[139] Billings, JJ. Ovulation method of family planning. *Lancet*, 1972, 2 (7788), 1193-1194.

[140] Billings, JJ. The validation of the Billings ovulation method by laboratory research and field trials. *Acta Europaea Fertilitatis*, 1981, 22 (1), 9-15.

[141] Brown, JB; Blackwell, LF; Billings, JJ; Conway, B; Cox RI; Garrett, G; Holmes, J;. Smithe, MA Natural family planning. *Am J Obstet Gynecol,* 1987, 157 (4 Pt 2), 1062-1069.

[142] Giacchi, E; Saporosi, A; Leone, E; De Marinis, L; Pontecorvi, A; Bompiani, A; Mancini, A. Subclinical hypothyroidism and ovarian function: diagnostic value of the Billing's ovulation method. *Abstracts of the XIX World Congress on Fertility & Sterility, IFFS (International Federation of Fertility Societies),* Durban, South Africa, april 29-may 3, 2007, p. 125 (abstract).

[143] Giacchi, E; Saporosi, A; Milardi, D; Merola, AM; Pellicanò, P; Squintani, MC; De Marinis, L; Jensen, L ; Mancini, A. Infertility in luteal defect due to hypothyroidism. In: *IFFS 2001 Selected Free Communication,* Bologna:Monduzzi Editore, 2001, pp. 87-91.

[144] Ruder, EH; Hartman, TJ: Goldman, MB Impact of oxidative stress on female fertility. *Curr Opin Obstet Gynecol*, 2009, 21 (3), 219-22.

[145] Li, S; Washburn, KA; Moore, R; Uno, T; Teng, C; Nwebold, RR; McLachalan, JA; Negishi, M. Developmental exposure to diethylstilbestrol elicits demethylation of estrogen-responsive lactoferrin gene in mouse uterus. *Cancer Res*, 1997, 57(19), 4356-4359.

[146] Anway, MD; Cupp, AS; Uzumcu, M; Skinner MK. Epigenetic transgenerational actions of endocrine disruptors and male fertility. *Science*, 2005, 308(5727), 1466-1469.

[147] Ruder, EH; Hartman, TJ; Blumberg, J; Goldman, M.B. Oxidative stress and antioxidants: exposure and impact on female fertility. *Hum Reprod Update*, 2008, 14 (4), 345-357.

In: Hypothyroidism ISBN: 978-1-62618-872-3
Editors: A. O'Neill and M. R. Quinn

Chapter II

Age-based TSH Levels in the Hypothyroidism Treatment

A. B. Mañas-Martinez and J. A. Gimeno-Orna
Department of Endocrinology, Lozano-Blesa Hospital,
Zaragoza, Spain

Abstract

The goal of hypothyroidism treatment is restoration of the euthyroid state in all the tissues. Monitoring the adequacy of levothyroxine therapy is easily done by measuring the serum thyrotropin (TSH) levels. This measurement should be within the normal range.

The National Health and Nutrition Examinations Survey (NHANES) sampling attempts to represent the U.S. population. Data from NHANES indicates that in population with iodine sufficiency, the serum TSH levels increase with age. Furthermore, in people with no clinical or biochemical experience of thyroid disease, no change has been observed in free thyroxine (FT4) concentrations. Other results from cross-sectional studies have also found an increase in TSH with age in populations free of thyroid disease. Additionally the raised of TSH observed in people with exceptional longevity suggests that the change of thyroid axis could be protective.

Thus, it seems that there is a progressive shift in the serum TSH distribution curve toward higher TSH values with increasing age. Based on these results, some researchers recommend the adoption of age-specific reference ranges for TSH, however this remains a matter of debate.

This paper is aimed to review medical research supporting the use of age- specific TSH reference ranges and subsequently an age-related TSH target to treat hypothyroidism.

Introduction

The most common thyroid disorder in iodine sufficient populations is primary hypothyroidism.

The NHANES III [1], designed to give a statistics of the health and nutritional status of the non- institutionalized US population, showed that the prevalence of subclinical disease was 4.3% and of overt disease was 0.3%. In the British Whickham survey 9.3% of women and 1.2% of men had serum TSH values over 10 mIU/L [2].

In order to make the diagnosis of primary thyroid dysfunction the TSH level is the best screening test [3]. According to NHANES III [4], the upper limit of the TSH reference range is approximately 4.12 mIU/liter. A diagnosis of subclinical primary hypothyroidism (SH) is done with a TSH level above 4.12 mIU/liter and FT4 levels within the reference range.

There is a general agreement that patients with TSH levels above 10 mIU/liter must be treated; nevertheless there is no clear evidence about treating patients with TSH levels between 4.12-10 mIU/liter, except in the case of pregnant women.

In fact, there are virtually no clinical- trial outcome to support treating patients with SH [3, 5]. Moreover every subject has a unique thyroid axis function with specific set points for TSH [6]. Due to the prevalence of this thyroid dysfunction, it´s essential to set the TSH reference range properly in order to avoid unnecessary treatment with levothyroxine that might not provide benefit and could adversely affect the health of misclassified hypothyroid subjects [4].

On the same way a TSH target has to be defined in treated patients in order to achieve the best risk-benefit balance. The clinical question is: Should this TSH target be the same for all patients or should be modulated according to their age?

TSH Reference Range

1. Defining a TSH Reference Range

The TSH distribution curve appears to have a non-Gaussian shape on a linear scale due to its skewness toward higher TSH values. So the recommended analyses employ a log-transformed of TSH levels and define the reference range using the median and 95% confidence limits [9].

In the recent years, the TSH reference range, particularly the upper limit, has been a source of controversy due to its implications on diagnosis of SH and consequently the treatment with levothyroxine [8-9].

The NHANES III research has focused on 16,533 people who were classified as the disease-free population. They were not known to have diseases such as thyroid dysfunction or goiter. A reference population of 13,344 was created from the disease-free population, after excluding people who were recognized to have risk factors for thyroid dysfunction, such as having detectable thyroglobulin or thyroid peroxidase antibodies. The TSH 97.5th percentile for this population was 4.12 mIU/L [1]. Other analyses from these data used the TSH frequency distribution curves for the selected age deciles (from 20-29 year to 80 years and older). Similarities in the shape of the curves have been observed in the disease- free and reference populations. However, differences can be seen in their peak frequencies that were shifted toward higher TSH concentrations with age [8]. In fact, the 97.5th percentile was about 3.6 mIU/L in people aged between 20-30 and 5.9 and 7.5 mIU/L in those who were 70-79 and 80 years or older, respectively. Every 10 years increase in the subjects´ age could increase the TSH upper limit by 0.3 mIU/L [10].

If the increasing 50th and 97.5th percentiles noted with aging resulted simply from an increase in prevalence of hypothyroidism, the peak frequency would occur at the same TSH concentration than young individuals, and a larger skew toward higher values would be observed [4]. Nevertheless, the similarities in the shapes of the curves suggest that each group of age has its own TSH reference values. Therefore it could be desirable to create an age-based TSH reference range as the use of the same interval for all patients could result in misclassification [3,4,7,10]. The most obvious impact could be found on people above 85 years old [9].

On the other hand, other studies demonstrate that there is not difference in the TSH values among age groups [12,13]. However, it should be emphasized that in these studies the oldest group included people younger than 65 [12] and the elderly were underrepresented [13].

However, the apparent discrepancies may not be only to the age-difference of studied groups, but also to iodine supply, an important modifier of thyroid function. Consequently an inverse relationship between TSH and age has been seen in iodine deficient population without thyroid autoantibodies [14-16].

This has been explained by an increased prevalence of hyperthyroidism and nodularity among the oldest age groups.

It can be affirmed that reference serum TSH levels of every region [12-16], according to iodine supply, could not be comparable to the reference values that were established for the U.S. population [1]. The Hanford Thyroid Disease Study, in agreement with NHANES III, established that the 97.5th percentile for TSH by immunochemiluminometric assay (ICMA) is 4.1 mIU/L in iodine sufficient populations with no evidence of thyroid disease, including a normal thyroid ultrasound and negative thyroid autoantibodies [17].

2. Physiological Mechanisms Modulating TSH Levels with Age

The outcome of most studies indicates that TSH distribution curve shifts to the right with aging in iodine sufficient areas [1,4,10,11]. The scientists have tried to explain whether this phenomenon is intrinsic to aging or it´s modulated by other mechanisms [1, 4, 8-10,18,19].

There seems to be an "altered set point" of the hypothalamic-pituitary-thyroid axis with aging. This could arise from diminished sensitivity of thyrotropes to the negative feedback of thyroid hormones. Nevertheless it would be also accompanied by an increase in FT4 concentrations, something that was not observed in previous studies [18, 19]. An age-related reduction in TSH bioactivity could influence the TSH pattern curve. It is known that TSH exists in various isoforms, which generates a mixture of oligosaccharide structures with different bioactivity [20]. The shift in circulating TSH isoforms could either be facilitated or be a consequence of healthy aging. It is hypothesized that exceptional longevity might be linked with decreased thyroid hormone secretion associated with increasing serum TSH concentrations [21]. Thyroid hormone has profound impact on metabolic rate and body temperature in different ways, including modulating mitocondrial activity, membrane composition and ion permeability. The relationship between longevity and hypothyroidism is considered to lower levels of reactive oxygen species production and oxidative stress [22]. According to this theory, the age- related TSH distribution would be also verified in people with exceptional longevity. This has been well -determined not only in population of Ashkenazi Jews centenarians [19] and in nonagerian siblings [23] but also in centenarian Ashkenazi offsprings [24]. Moreover, it has been found that every individual has a unique thyroid function, with concentrations maintained within relatively narrow limits and with large variations among individuals [6]. This raises the idea that the thyroid function's set point between free hormones and TSH is genetically determined [19,24]. Therefore, not only a longer survival might be associated with an age- related increased TSH levels, but also it could be genetically determined partway.

On the other hand, another theory explaining this TSH distribution curve could be the presence of occult thyroid disease. However, this was not supported by a 13- years follow-up of 908 people without evidence of thyroid disease, in the Busselton Health Study [18]. It was observed that there was an increase of TSH levels of 0.32 mIU/L during the follow-up, whereas FT4 concentration was unchanged.

The greatest increase in TSH occurred in the oldest participants and in participants with lower baseline TSH values. If TSH levels had risen because of thyroid occult disease, the most increased levels should have be found in individuals in the upper part of the TSH population distribution and accompanied by a fall of FT4 levels. Unmodified FT4 levels have also been objectified in centenarians despite the increase in TSH values [19]. An additional consideration was reflected by the Cardiovascular Health Study [25]: resolution of subclinical hypothyroidism was common in subjects aged older than 65 with a TSH of 4.5–6.9 mIU/L (46 %). This suggests that the use of a unique set of thyroid function test might lead to misclassification.

Usefulness of Subclinical Hypothyroidism Treatment

The threshold levels of TSH for treatment of SH in non-pregnant individuals has been controversial. Data on the association with coronary heart disease (CHD), cardiovascular disease (CVD) and total mortality are conflicting among observational studies.

1. Benefits of Treatment

As recently revised by Franklyn et al [26], it has been indicated that SH is associated with minor cholesterol elevations, left ventricular diastolic dysfunction, systemic vascular resistance and arterial thickness. However, epidemiological studies of vascular morbidity and mortality have shown inconsistent results.

Several years ago, the Rotterdam Study [27] reported that SH might be involved in the pathogenesis of up to 14 % of all myocardial infarctions. A 20-years follow-up of the Whickham cohort [28] showed that participants with SH had an increased risk of incident CHD (HR=1.76; 95% CI 1.15-2.71) and incident CHD mortality (HR=1.79; 95% CI 1.02-3.56). Recently, baseline SH was associated with a statistically significant increased risk of CHD mortality (HR=1.38; 95% CI 1.03-1.84) in the Scandinavian HUNT Study [29], that included 26707 participants followed-up during 12 years.

On the other hand, there´s some evidence suggesting that SH is neither linked with higher cardiovascular risk nor mortality. In people aged older than 65, a single measurement of thyroid function did not predict total or cause-specific mortality in the MrOS study [30]. Besides, in subjects aged older than 85 and living in Leiden [31], increasing levels of TSH and decreasing levels of FT4, both representing a decrease of thyroid function, were associated with a survival benefit.

More information is derived from three meta-analysis. In the first one [32], that included 11 prospective cohort studies, with 542494 person-years of follow-up, the risk of CHD and CHD mortality increased with higher TSH levels. TSH levels between 7-10 mIU/L or above were associated statistically significant with an increased CHD mortality risk (HR=1.42 and HR=1.58 respectively).

The second remarkable meta-analysis [33] included studies with individuals with TSH below 10 mIU/L. The prognosis of CVD mortality was assessed in 8 longitudinal studies (1417 people with SCH and 13302 euthyroid participants) where an age-based heterogeneity risk conferred by SH was found. CVD mortality was increased in studies including individuals younger than 65 (OR=1.37; 95%CI 1.04-1.79) whereas nor such risk was evident in the studies with subjects aged older than 65 (OR=0.85; 95%CI 0.56-1.29).

A third meta-analysis [34] investigated the association between SH and heart failure and concluded that risk was increased with TSH above 10 mIU/L. However, a significant trend across age categories was not found.

It is clear that well-designed randomized control trials of treatment of SH are needed to investigate if CVD risk can be reduced, but any of these trials needs to consider the age of the participants. Currently, the best evidence to ascertain the usefulness of SH treatment can be inferred from the United Kingdom General Practitioner Research Database [5]. Individuals aged 40 or older, with a first-ever increased TSH level of 5 - 10 mIU/L and normal FT4 levels, were evaluated. The participants aged 40-70 and those older than 70 were considered separately to calculate the CHD risk, due to statistically significant interaction. Time-dependent levothyroxine treatment was associated with lower CHD events (HR=0.61; 95% CI 0.39-0.95) and all cause mortality (HR=0.36; 95% CI 0.19-0.66) in the younger group, but not in the older group.

2. Risks of Treatment

Several studies show that approximately 40% of patients treated with levothyroxine have subsequent serum TSH concentrations outside the reference range [35]. Hence, the decision to treat the SH may not frequently lead to ideal biochemical control. In our experience (unpublished observations) only 69% of treated patients have a TSH level between 0.45 and 4.12 mIU/L.

Overtreatment leading to subclinical hyperthyroidism could be detrimental for the patient. As revised by Cooper and Biondi [36], this condition is associated with an increased frequency of premature atrial and ventricular beats, atrial fibrillation and risk of fracture. Using the TEARS dataset of Scotland, Flynn et al [37] analyzed the CVD and fracture risks in patients receiving a long-term replacement treatment with levothyroxine.

It was also evaluated what level of TSH concentration might be safe. Each patient´s time-weighted geometric mean (back transformed mean of the logarithmic values) TSH (mIU/L) was classified as suppressed (<0.03), low (0.04-0.4), normal (0.4-4) and high (>4). The best fit for both CVD and fracture was a second-degree fractional polynomial, with the highest level of risk associated with extreme levels of TSH concentrations. A suppressed TSH level increased CVD risk (HR=1.37; 95% CI 1.17-1.60), dysrhythmia risk (HR=1.60; 95% CI 1.10-2.33) and osteoporotic fracture risk (HR=2.02; 95% CI 1.55-2.62).

Conclusion

Evidence suggests that TSH reference range is age-dependent, with higher values in the older individuals and it´s probably associated with a survival benefit. Subclinical hypothyroidism increases CVD mortality risk only in people under the age of 65. A benefit of levothyroxine therapy in SH with TSH levels between 5 and 10 mIU/L has only been demonstrated in patients under the age of 70. Besides overtreatment is not unusual, which is also associated with an increase of CVD and fracture risks.

Current guidelines [3] recommend treating all patients with SH and TSH levels higher than 10 mIU/L and treating patients with TSH levels between 4.12 and 10 mIU/L on a selective way. We think that in this last SH group, the treatment is mostly justifiable in people under the age of 70. Moreover, the TSH serum concentrations in the treatment with levothyroxine might be adjusted higher in patients above the age of 70, to mimic physiological values and decrease the over-treatment risk. We agree with Cooper´s [36] recommendation for older patients: a TSH target between 4 and 6 mIU/L.

However, a definitive evidence for optimal TSH targets can only come from a well-designed, randomized placebo-controlled clinical trial.

References

[1] Hollowell, JG; Staehling, NW; Flanders, WD; Hannon, WH; Gunter, EW; Spencer, CA; Braverman, LE. Serum TSH, T (4), and thyroid antibodies in the United States population (1988 to 1994): National Health and Nutrition Examination Survey (NHANES III). *J Clin Endocrinol Metab, 2002*, 87, 489–499.

[2] Vanderpump, MP; Tunbridge, WM; French, JM; Appleton, D; Bates, D; Clark, F; Grimley Evans, J; Hasan, DM; Rodgers, H; Tunbridge, F; Young, ET. The incidence of thyroid disorders in the community: a twenty-year follow-up of the Whickham Survey. *Clin Endocrinol,* 1995, 43, 55–68.

[3] Garber, JR; Cobin, RH; Gharib, H; Hennessey, JV; Klein, I; Mechanick, JI; Pessah-Pollack, R; Singer, PA; Woebe, KA. Clinical Practice Guidelines for Hypothyroidism in Adults: Cosponsored by the American

Association of Clinical Endocrinologists and the American Thyroid Association. *Thyroid,* 2012, 22, 1200- 1235.

[4] Surks, MI; Hollowell, JG. Age- Specific distribution of serum thyrotropin and antithyroid antiboides in the US population: Implications for the prevalence of subclinical hypothyroidism. *J Clin Endocrinol Metab,* 2007, 92, 4575- 4582.

[5] Razvi S, Weaver JU, Butler TJ, Pearce SH. Levothyroxine treatment of subclinical hypothyroidism, fatal and nonfatal cardiovascular events, and mortality. *Arch Intern Med,* 2012,172, 811-817.

[6] Rozing, MP; Houwing-Duistermaat, JJ; Slagboom, PE; Beekman, M; Frölich, M; de Craen, AJ; Westendorp, RG; van Heemst, D. Familial Longevity is Associated with Decreased Thyroid Function. *J Clin Endocrinol Metab,* 2010, 95,4979–4984.

[7] Boucai, L; Surks, MI. Reference limits of serum TSH and free T4 are significantly influenced by race and age in an urban outpatient medical practice. *Clin Endocrinol,* 2009, 70, 788-793.

[8] Braban, G; Beck- Peccoz, P; Jarzab, B; Laurberg, P; Orgiazzi, J; Szabolcs, I; Weetman, AP; Wiersinga, WM. Is there a need to redefine the upper normal limit of TSH? *Eur J Endocrinol,* 2006, 154, 633- 637.

[9] Sucks, MI;Goswami, G;Daniels, GH. The thyrotropin reference range should remain unchanged. *J Clin Endocrinol Metab,* 2005, 90, 5489-5496.

[10] Boucai, L; Hollowell, JG; Surks, MI. An approach for development of age, gender and ethnicity- specific thyrotropin reference limits. *Thyroid,* 2011, 21, 5- 11.

[11] Kahapola- Arachchige, K; Hadlow, N; Wardrop, R; Lim, Ee; Walsh, JP. Age- specific TSH reference ranges have minimal impact on the diagnosis of thyroid dysfunction. *Clin Endocrinol,* 2012, 77, 773- 779.

[12] Knudsen, N; Bülow, I; Jorgensen, T; Laurberg, P; Ovesen, L; Perrild, H. Comparative study of thyroid function and types of thyroid dysfunction in two areas in Denmark with slightly different iodine status. *Eur J Endocrinol,* 2000, 143, 485- 491

[13] Chenyan, L; Haixia, G; Xiaochun, T; Lai, Y; Chen, Y; Yu, J; Li, N; Wang, B; Jiang, F; Wang, J; Fan, C; Wang, H; Zhang, H; Teng, W; Shan, Z. An epidemiological study of the serum thyrotropin reference range and factors that influence serum thyrotropin levels in iodine sufficient areas of China. *Endocr J,* 2011, 58, 995- 1002.

[14] Kratzsch, J; Fiedler, GM;Leichtle, A; Brügel, M; Buchbinder, S; Otto, L; Sabri, O; Matthes, G; Thiery, J. New reference intervals for thyrotropin

and thyroid hormones based on national academy of clinical biochemistry criteria and regular ultrasonography of the thyroid. *Clin Chem,* 2005, 51, 1480- 1486

[15] Guan, H; Shan, Z; Teng, X; Li, Y; Teng, D; Jin, Y; Yu, X; Fan, C; Chong, W; Yang, F; Dai, H; Yu, Y; Li, J; Chen, Y; Zhao, D; Shi, X; Hu, F; Mao, J; Gu, X; Yang, R; Chen, W; Tong, Y; Wang, W; Gao, T; Li, C; Teng, W. Influence of iodine on the reference interval of TSH and the optimal interval of TSH: results of a follow- up study in areas with different iodine intakes. *Clin Endocrinol,* 2008, 69, 13- 141.

[16] Völzke, H; Alte, D; Kohlmann, T; Lüdemann, J; Nauck, M; John, U; Meng, W. Reference intervals of serum thyroid function tests in a previously iodine-deficient area. *Thyroid,* 2005, 15, 279-85.

[17] Hamilton TE; Davis S; Onstad L; Kopecky KJ. Thyrotropin Levels in a population with no clinical, autoantibody, or ultrasonographic evidence of thyroid disease: implications for the diagnosis of subclinical hypothyroidism. *J Clin Endocrinol Metab,* 2008, 93, 1224-1230.

[18] Bremner, AP; Feddema, P; Leedman, PJ; Brown, SJ; Beilby JP; Lim, EM; Wilson, SG; O'Leary, PC; Walsh, JP. Age- related changes in thyroid function: a longitudinal study of a community- based cohort. *J Clin Endocrinol Metab,* 2012, 97, 1554- 1562.

[19] Atzmon, G; Barzilai, N; Hollowell, JG; Surks, MI; Gabriely, I. Extreme longevity is associated with increased serum thyrotropin. *J Clin Endocrinol Metab,* 2009,94, 1251–1254.

[20] Hulbert, AJ; Pamplona, R; Buffenstetin, R; Buttemer, WA. Life and death: metabolic rate, membrane composition, and lifespan of animals. *Physiol Rev,* 2007, 87, 1175- 1213.

[21] Szkudlinski, MW; Fremont, V; Ronin, C; Weintraub, BD. Thyroid-Stimulating Hormone and Thyroid-Stimulating Hormone Receptor Structure-Function Relationships. *Physiol Rev,* 2002, 82, 473- 502.

[22] Speakman, JR; Selman, C; McLaren, JS; Harper, EJ. Living fast, dying when? The link between aging and energetics. *J Nutr,* 2002, 132, 1538-1597.

[23] Rozing, MP; Houwing- Duistermaat, JJ; Slagboom, PE; Beekman, M; Frölich, M; de Craen, AJ; Westendorp, RG; van Heemst, D. Familial Longevity is Associated with Decreased Thyroid function. *J Clin Endocrinol Metab,* 2010, 95, 4979- 4984.

[24] Atzmon, G; Barzilai, N; Surks, MI; Gabriely, I. Genetic predisposition to elevated serum thyrotropin is associated with exceptional longevity. *J Clin Endocrinol Metab,* 2009; 94, 4768- 4775.

[25] Somwaru, LL; Rariy, CM; Arnold, AM; Cappola, AR. The Natural History of Subclinical Hypothyroidism in the Elderly: The Cardiovascular Health Study. *J Clin Endocrinol Metab,* 2012, 97, 1962-1969.

[26] Franklyn JA. The thyroid – too much and too little across the ages. The consequences of subclinical thyroid dysfunction. *Clin Endocrinol,* 2013, 78, 1-8.

[27] Hak, AE; Pols, HAP; Visser, TJ; Drexhage, HA; Hofman, A; Witteman, JCM. Subclinical hypothyroidism is an independent risk factor for atherosclerosis and myocardial infarction in elderly women: the Rotterdam study. *Ann Intern Med,* 2000,132, 270-278.

[28] Razvi, S; Weaver, JU; Vanderpump, MP; Pearce SHS. The incidence of ischemic heart disease and mortality in people with subclinical hypothyroidism: reanalysis of the Whickham Survey Cohort. *J Clin Endocrinol Metab,* 2010, 95, 1734-1740.

[29] Asvold, BO; Bjoro, T; Platou, C; Vatten, LJ. Thyroid function and the risk of coronary heart disease: 12-year follow-up of the HUNT Study in Norway. *Clin Endocrinol,* 2012, 77, 911-917.

[30] Waring, AC; Harrison, S; Samuels, MH; Ensrud, KE; LeBlanc, ES; Hoffman, AR; Orwoll, E; Fink, HA; Barret-Connor, E; Bauer, DC. Thyroid function and mortality in older men: a prospective study. *J Clin Endocrinol Metab,* 2012, 97, 862-870.

[31] Gussekloo, J; Van Exel, E; De Craen, AJ; Meinders, AE; Frölich, M; Westendorp, RT. Thyroid status, disability and cognitive function and survival in old age. *JAMA,* 2004, 292, 2591- 2599.

[32] Rodondi, N; den Elzen, WP; Bauer, DC; Cappola, AR; Razvi, S; Walsh, JP; Asvold, BO; Lervasi, G; Imaizumi, M; Collet, TH; Bremner, A; Maisonneuve, P; Sgarbi, JA; Khaw, KT; Vanderpump, MP; Newman, AB; Cornuz, J; Franklyn, JA; Westendorp, RG; Vittinghoff, E; Gussekloo, J; Subclinical Hypothyroidism and the Risk of Coronary Heart Disease and Mortality. *JAMA,* 2010, 304, 1365- 1374.

[33] Razvi, S; Shakoor, A; Vanderpump, M; Weaver, JU; Pearce, SH. The Influence of Age on the Relationship between Subclinical Hypothyroidism and Ischemic Heart Disease: A Metaanalysis. *Clin Endocrinol Metab,* 2008, 93, 2998–3007

[34] Gencer, B; Collet, TH; Virgini, V; Bauer, DC; Gusselkloo, J; Cappola, AR; Nanchen, D; den Elzen, WPJ; Balmer, P; Luben, RN; Iacoviello, M; Triggiani, V; Cornuz, J; Newman, AB; Khaw, KT; Jukema, JW; Westendorp, RGJ; Vittinghoff, E; Aujesky, D; Rodondi, N. Subclinical

thyroid dysfunction and the risk of heart failure events: an individual participant data analysis from six prospective cohorts. *Circulation,* 2012, 126,1040–1049.

[35] Canaris, GJ; Manowitz, NR; Mayor, G; Ridgway, EC. The Colorado thyroid disease prevalence study. Arch Intern Med, 2000, 160, 526-534.

[36] Cooper, DS; Biondi, B. Subclinical thyroid disease. *Lancet,* 2012, 379, 1142-1154.

[37] Flynn, RW; Bonellie, SR; Jung, RT; MacDonald, TM; Morris, AD; Leese, GP. Serum thyroid-stimulating hormone concentration and morbidity from cardiovascular disease and fractures in patients on long-term thyroxine therapy. *J Clin Endocrinol Metab,* 2010, 95, 186-193.

In: Hypothyroidism
Editors: A. O'Neill and M. R. Quinn
ISBN: 978-1-62618-872-3

Chapter III

Overt Hypothyroidism, Subclinical Hypothyroidism and Isolated Hypothyroxinemia during Pregnancy: New Guidelines

Baha Zantour *

Department of Endocrinology, Tahar Sfar Hospital, Mahdia, Tunisia

Abstract

Thyroid dysfunction is common during gestation. The prevalence of hypothyroidism during pregnancy is estimated to be 0.3-0.5% for overt hypothyroidism (OH) and 2-3% for subclinical hypothyroidism (SCH). The prevalence of isolated hypothyroxinemia is 1-2% in sufficient iodine intake regions. Chronic autoimmune thyroiditis is the main cause of hypothyroidism during pregnancy, apart from iode deficiency.

Reference ranges for thyroid function tests differ in healthy pregnant women from those of healthy non pregnant women. A TSH of 2.5 mIU/l is now accepted as the upper limit of normal for TSH in the first trimester. OH is defined as an elevated TSH (>2.5 mIU/l) in conjunction

* Corresponding author mail: bahazantour@yahoo.fr.

with a decreased free T4 (FT4) concentration. Women with TSH levels of 10.0 mIU/l or above, irrespective of their FT4 levels are also considered to have OH. SCH is defined as a serum TSH between 2.5 and 10.0 mIU/l with a normal FT4 concentration. Isolated hypothyroxinemia is defined as a normal maternal TSH concentration in conjunction with FT4 concentrations in the lower 5th or 10th percentile of the reference range.

It is now well established that OH is associated with an increased risk of adverse pregnancy complications, as well as detrimental effects upon fetal neurocognitive development. However, data regarding SCH and maternal isolated hypothyroxinemia are controversial.

In the past several years, there has been considerable discussion about whether all pregnant women should be screened in order to identify and treat thyroid dysfunction. To date there are not enough data for or against universal screening. In their recent guidelines, the American Thyroid Association and the Endocrine Society recommend prenatal measurement of serum TSH in women at high risk for thyroid illness on the basis of their medical history, physical exam, or prior chemical data.

Women with preexisting hypothyroidism will need to increase their prepregnancy dose of thyroxine to maintain a normal thyroid function. In a newly diagnosed hypothyroid patient, a full replacement thyroxine dose should be instituted immediately and thyroxine dosage adjusted on the base of results of thyroid function tests. Serum FT4 level should be at the upper end of normal range for each trimester of pregnancy, serum TSH level should be < 2.5 mIU/L in the first trimester or 3 mIU/l in the second and third trimesters. Since maternal morbidity as well as prenatal morbidity and consequences on the neuropsychological development of the child have been reported in subclinical hypothyroidism, most guidelines recommend thyroxine replacement in women with subclinical hypothyroidism. Management of isolated hypothyroxinemia during pregnancy is controversial and requires further study.

Thyroid dysfunction is common during gestation. The prevalence of hypothyroidism during pregnancy is estimated to be 0.3-0.5% for overt hypothyroidism (OH) and 2-3% for subclinical hypothyroidism (SCH). The prevalence of isolated hypothyroxinemia is 1-2% in sufficient iodine intake regions. Chronic autoimmune thyroiditis is the main cause of hypothyroidism during pregnancy, apart from iode deficiency [1, 2].

Knowledge regarding the interaction between the thyroid and pregnancy is advancing at a rapid pace. In this context, the American Thyroid Association ATA [3] and the Endocrine Society ES [4] reviewed existing guidelines according to recent knowledge and published their practical guidelines in 2011 and 2012 respectively on management of thyroid dysfunction during pregnancy and postpartum.

Thyroid function test results of healthy pregnant women differ from those of healthy non pregnant women. During pregnancy, women have lower serum TSH concentrations than before pregnancy. Most studies also report a substantial decrease in serum free T4 (FT4) concentrations with progression of gestation [4, 5]. Both ATA and ES recommend caution in the interpretation of serum FT4 levels during pregnancy, and that each laboratory should establish trimester-specific reference ranges for pregnant women if using a FT4 assay. The ATA precise that the optimal method to assess serum FT4 during pregnancy is measurement of T4 in the dialysate or ultrafiltrate of serum samples employing on-line extraction/liquid chromatography/tandem mass spectrometry (LC/MS/MS) [3]. This assay technology, unfortunately, is currently not widely available due to high instrument and operating costs. In the ES guidelines, the non-pregnant total T4 (TT4) range (5-12 μg/dL or 50-150 nmol/L) can be adapted in the second and third trimesters by multiplying this range by 1.5-fold. Alternatively, the FT4 index ("adjusted T4 ") appears to be a reliable assay during pregnancy [4]. FT4 index is calculated by TT4 x T3 uptake or a ratio of TT4 and thyroxine binding globulin, but trimester-specific reference intervals for FT4 index have not been established in a reference population [3]. The ATA considers that serum TSH is a more accurate indication of thyroid status in pregnancy than any of these alternative methods. If trimester-specific reference ranges for TSH are not available in the laboratory, the following reference ranges are recommended: first trimester, 0.1–2.5 mIU/L; second trimester, 0.2–3.0 mIU/L; third trimester, 0.3–3.0 mIU/L [3].

OH is defined as an elevated TSH (>2.5 mIU/L) in conjunction with a decreased FT4 concentration. Women with TSH levels of 10.0 mIU/L or above, irrespective of their FT4 levels are also considered to have OH. SCH is defined as a serum TSH between 2.5 and 10.0 mIU/L with a normal FT4 concentration [3]. Isolated hypothyroxinemia is defined during pregnancy as a normal maternal TSH concentration in conjunction with FT4 concentrations in the lower 5th or 10th percentile of the reference range [3].

Although it is now well established that OH is associated with an increased risk of adverse pregnancy complications, as well as detrimental effects upon fetal neurocognitive development [6], data regarding SCH [6, 7] and maternal isolated hypothyroxinemia are controversial [8, 9]. Maternal hypothyroidism should be avoided [4]. The recommended treatment of maternal hypothyroidism is the administration of oral Levothyroxine (LT4). It is strongly recommended not to use other thyroid preparations such as T3 or desiccated thyroid [3]. If hypothyroidism has been diagnosed before pregnancy, ES and ATA recommend adjustment of the preconception thyroxine dose to reach prior to pregnancy a TSH level not higher than 2.5 mIU/L [3, 4]. Treated hypothyroid patients (receiving LT4), who are newly pregnant should independently increase their dose of LT4 by 25%–30% upon a missed menstrual cycle or positive home pregnancy test and notify their caregiver promptly [3, 4]. One means of accomplishing this adjustment is to increase LT4 from once daily dosing to a total of nine doses per week (29% increase) [3, 4]. In the ATA guidelines, they recognize that there exists great interindividual variability regarding the increased amount of LT4 necessary to maintain a normal TSH throughout pregnancy, with some women requiring only 10%–20% increased dosing, while others may require as much as an 80% increase [3]. The etiology of maternal hypothyroidism, as well as the preconception level of TSH, may provide insight into the magnitude of necessary LT4 increase. Clinicians should seek this information upon assessment of the patient after pregnancy is confirmed [3]. ES guidelines recommend that all women receiving LT4 should be verbally screened before conception to assess their understanding of changing LT4 requirements following conception. These women should be counseled to contact a physician or medical professional immediately upon a missed menstrual cycle or suspicion of pregnancy to check their serum TSH level [4]. In pregnant patients with treated hypothyroidism, maternal TSH should be checked at least once between 26 and 32 weeks gestation [3]. After delivery, most hypothyroid women need to decrease the LT4 dosage they received during pregnancy to the pre-pregnancy dose [3, 4].

If overt hypothyroidism is diagnosed during pregnancy, thyroid function tests should be normalized as rapidly as possible. LT4 dosage should be titrated to rapidly reach and thereafter maintain serum TSH concentrations of less than 2.5 mI/L in the first trimester (or 3 mIU/L in second and third trimester) or to trimester-specific TSH ranges. Thyroid function tests should be re-measured within 30-40 days [4].

Guidelines regarding SCH are less unanimous. SCH may be associated with an adverse outcome for both the mother and offspring [10, 11]. There is a single randomized controlled trial that demonstrated that LT4 intervention at 9 weeks gestation resulted in a reduction in adverse pregnancy outcomes in TPO antibodies (TPOAb) positive women with SCH [12]. In the ATA guidelines, they distinguish two situations: Women who have SCH and are positive for TPOAb should be treated with LT4. However, there is insufficient evidence to recommend for or against universal LT4 treatment in TPOAb negative pregnant women with SCH [3]. The ES recommends LT4 replacement in women with SCH regardless the positivity for TPOAb, given that the potential benefits outweigh the potential risks [4].

Studies on isolated hypothyroxinemia are few and data are controversial. In some studies, infants and toddlers whose mothers had isolated maternal hypothyroxinemia during gestation (12 to 20 weeks) had lower mean intelligence, psychomotor, or behavioral scores compared with children born to women with normal thyroid function during gestation [9]. In another study, risks of adverse pregnancy outcomes were not increased in over 200 pregnant women with isolated hypothyroxinemia [8]. To date, no randomized, interventional trial of LT4 therapy has been performed in pregnant women with isolated hypothyroxinemia. So, the ATA guidelines do not recommend therapy for such women at present [3]. However, in the opinion of the committee of the ES, partial replacement therapy may be initiated at the discretion of the caregiver, with continued monitoring [4].

In euthyroid women who are TPOAb positive prior to conception, both OH and SCH may occur during the stress of pregnancy as the ability of the thyroid to augment production is compromised and increasing demand outstrips supply. When this happens, an elevated TSH occurs [13]. In these women, both ES and ATA recommend monitoring for elevation of TSH above the normal range for pregnancy [3, 4]. The ATA recommends that serum TSH should be evaluated every 4 weeks during the first half of pregnancy and at least once between 26 and 32 weeks gestation [3]. The ES recommends screening for serum TSH abnormalities before pregnancy, as well as during the 1st and 2nd trimesters of pregnancy [4]. Multiple observational studies [14, 15, 16] and 2 meta-analyses [17, 18] have confirmed a 2-4 fold risk of miscarriage among euthyroid TPOAb positive women, compared to euthyroid TPOAb negative women. Some studies [19, 20] but not all [21, 22], have also found associations between thyroid autoimmunity and increased rates of recurrent miscarriage. The presence of maternal thyroid antibodies has also been associated with elevated risk for premature delivery [23] and postpartum thyroiditis [24]. Moreover, the positivity for thyroid autoantibodies in euthyroid pregnant women affects neuropsychological development of the offspring per se [25]. Only one randomized interventional trial with thyroxine treatment has suggested a decrease in the first trimester miscarriage rate in euthyroid antibody-positive women, but treatment duration was very brief before the outcome of interest [23]. The ES considers that universal screening for anti-thyroid antibodies, and possible treatment, cannot be recommended at this time [4]. Similarly, the ATA considers that there is insufficient evidence to recommend for or against screening all women for antithyroid antibodies in the first trimester of pregnancy nor to recommend for or against LT4 therapy in thyroid Ab positive euthyroid women during pregnancy [3].

In the past several years, there has been considerable discussion about whether all pregnant women should be screened in order to identify and treat thyroid dysfunction. Both OH and SCH are prevalent, SCH may be asymptomatic. Serum TSH is relatively inexpensive, widely available and is a reliable test in pregnancy, assuming that trimester-specific reference ranges are applied. However, it's not demonstrated that identification of SCH results in a beneficial intervention. The lack of high quality randomized controlled trials had led to mixed viewpoints among members of the ATA [3] and the ES [4]. Finally, both published in their guidelines that universal screening of healthy women for thyroid dysfunction before pregnancy is not recommended [3, 4]. The ATA agrees that there is insufficient evidence to recommend for or against universal TSH screening at the first trimester visit [3]. The committee of the ES could not reach agreement with regard to screening recommendations of all newly pregnant women for serum TSH.

Some members recommended screening of all pregnant women for serum TSH abnormalities by the 9th week or at the time of their first visit. Some members recommended neither for nor against universal screening of all pregnant women for TSH abnormalities at the time of their first visit.

Table 1. Recommended patient profiles for targeted thyroid disease case finding in women seeking pregnancy, or newly pregnant [4]

- Women over age 30 years
- Women with a family history or autoimmune thyroid disease or hypothyroidism
- Women with a goiter
- Women with thyroid antibodies, primarily thyroid peroxidase antibodies
- Women with symptoms or clinical signs suggestive of thyroid hypofunction
- Women with type 1 diabetes mellitus, or other autoimmune disorders
- Women with infertility
- Women with a prior history of preterm delivery
- Women with prior therapeutic head or neck irradiation or prior thyroid surgery
- Women currently receiving levothyroxine replacement

These members strongly support aggressive case finding to identify and test high-risk women (Table 1) for elevated TSH concentrations by the 9th week or at the time of their first visit before and during pregnancy, and recognize that in some situations, ascertainment of the individual's risk status may not be feasible. In such cases, and where the local practice environment is appropriate, testing of all women by 9 weeks of pregnancy or at the first prenatal visit is reasonable [4]. The ATA recognizes also that serum TSH values should be obtained early in pregnancy in women at high risk for overt OH. The recommended patient profiles for targeted thyroid disease case finding indicated by the ATA are those mentioned by the ES, morbid obesity (BMI _40 kg/m2), use of amiodarone or lithium, recent administration of iodinated radiologic contrast, infertility, and residing in an area of known moderate to severe iodine sufficiency [3].

Because no studies to date have demonstrated a benefit to treatment of isolated maternal hypothyroximenia, the ATA doesn't recommend universal FT4 screening of pregnant women [3].

Conclusion

Over the last decade, there has been a rapid expansion of knowledge regarding thyroid disease and pregnancy. Given the rapidity of advances in this field, it is not surprising that controversy surrounds optimal detection and management of thyroid disease in the pregnant woman. Recently, some prospective randomized studies have begun to produce critically needed data on the impact of treating thyroid disease on the pregnancy and the fetus. However, in developing the guidelines, the task forces created by the ES or the ATA faced the problem of the paucity of high quality double-blind placebo controlled trials in the field of thyroid and pregnancy. Such trials are needed to develop good evidence-based guidelines. Areas for future research include screening and treatment of SCH, isolated hypothyroxinemia and TPO Ab positivity in euthyroid pregnant women.

References

[1] Abalovich M, Amino N, Barbour L. A, Cobin R. H, Degroot L. J, Glinoer D, Mandel S. J, Stagnaro-Green A. Management of thyroid

dysfunction during pregnancy and postpartum: an Endocrine Society Clinical Practice Guideline. *Journal of Clinical Endocrinology and Metabolism* 2007; 92 (8 suppl): S1-47.

[2] Krassas G. E, Popper K, Glinoer D. Thyroid function and human reproductive health. *Endocrine Reviews* 2010; 31(5): 702-755.

[3] Stagnaro-Green A, Abalovich M, Alexander E, Azizi F, Mestman J, Negro R, Nixon A, Pearce EN, Soldin OP, Sullivan S, Wiersing W. Guidelines of the American Thyroid Association for the diagnosis and management of thyroid disease during pregnancy and postpartum. *Thyroid* 2011; 21(10): 1081-1125.

[4] De Groot L, Abalovich M, Alexander E. K, Amino N, Barbour L, Cobin R, Eastman C, Lazarus J, Luton D, Mandel S, Mestman J, Rovet J, Sullivan S. Management of thyroid dysfunction during pregnancy and postpartum: An Endocrine Society Clinical Practice Guideline. *Journal of Clinical Endocrinology and Metabolism* 2012; 97(8): 2543-2565.

[5] Soldin O. P, Soldin D, Sastoque M. Gestation-specific thyroxine and thyroid stimulating hormone levels in the United States and worldwide. *Therapeutic Drug Monitoring* 2007; 29(5); 553-559.

[6] Haddow J. E, Palomaki G. E, Allan W. C, Williams J. R, Knight G. J, Gagnon J, O'Heir C. E, Mitchell M. L, Hermos R. J, Waisbren S. E, Faix J. D, Klein R. Z. Maternal thyroid deficiency during pregnancy and subsequent neuropsychological development of the child. *New England Journal of Medicine* 1999; 341(8): 549-555.

[7] Casey B. M, Dashe J. S, Wells C. E, McIntire D. D, Byrd W, Leveno K. J, Cunningham F. G. Subclinical hypothyroidism and pregnancy outcomes. *Obstetrical Gynecology* 2005; 105(2): 239-215.

[8] Casey B. M, Dashe J. S, Spong C. Y, McIntire D. D, Leveno K. J, Cunningham G. F. Perinatal significance of isolated maternal hypothyroxinemia identified in the first half of pregnancy. *Obstetrical Gynecology* 2007; 109(5):1129-1135.

[9] Vermiglio F, Lo Presti V. P, Moleti M, Sidoti M, Tortorella G, Scaffidi G, Castagna M. G, Mattina F, Violi M. A, Crisà A, Artemisia A, Trimarchi F. Attention deficit and hyperactivity disorders in the offspring of mothers exposed to mild-moderate iodine deficiency: A possible novel iodine deficiency disorder in developed countries. *Journal of Clinical Endocrinology and Metabolism* 2004; 89(12): 6054–6060.

[10] Pop V. J, Kuijpens J. L, van Baar A. L, Verkerk G, van Son M. M, de Vijlder J. J, Vulsma T, Wiersinga W. M, Drexhage H. A, Vader H. L.

Low maternal free thyroxine concentrations during early pregnancy are associated with impaired psychomotor development in infancy. *Clinical Endocrinology* (Oxf) 1999; 50(2): 149–155.

[11] Wang S, Teng W. P, Li J. X, Wang W. W, Shan Z. Y. Effects of maternal subclinical hypothyroidism on obstetrical outcomes during early pregnancy. *Journal of Endocrinological Investigation* 2012; 35(3):322-325.

[12] Negro R, Schwartz A, Gismoudi R, Tinelli A, Mangieri T, Stagnaro-Green A. Universal screening versus case finding for detection and treatment of thyroid hormonal dysfunction during pregnancy. *Journal of Clinical Endocrinology and Metabolism* 2010; 95(4): 1699-1707.

[13] Glinoer D, Riahi M, Grun J. P, Kinthaert J. Risk of subclinical hypothyroidism in pregnant women with asymptomatic autoimmune thyroid disorders. *Journal of Clinical Endocrinology and Metabolism* 1994; 79:197–204.

[14] Abbassi-Ghanavati M, Casey B. M, Spong C. Y, McIntire D. D, Halvorson L. M, Cunningham F. G. Pregnancy outcomes in women with thyroid peroxidase antibodies. *Obstetrics Gynecology* 2010; 116(2 Pt 1): 381–386.

[15] Bagis T, Gokcel A, Saygili E. S. Autoimmune thyroid disease in pregnancy and the postpartum period: relationship to spontaneous abortion. *Thyroid* 2001;11(11):1049–1053.

[16] Glinoer D, Soto M. F, Bourdoux P, Lejeune B, Delange F, Lemone M, Kinthaert J, Robijn C, Grun J. P, de Nayer P. Pregnancy in patients with mild thyroid abnormalities: maternal and neonatal repercussions. *Journal of Clinical Endocrinology and Metabolism* 1991;73(2):421–427.

[17] Thangaratinam S, Tan A, Knox E, Kilby M. D, Franklyn J, Coomarasamy A. Association between thyroid autoantibodies and miscarriage and preterm birth: meta-analysis of evidence. *British Medical Journal* 2011; 342:d2616.

[18] Prummel M. F, Wiersinga W. M. Thyroid autoimmunity and miscarriage. *European Journal of Endocrinology* 2004;150(6):751–755.

[19] De Carolis C, Greco E, Guarino M. D, Perricone C, Dal Lago A, Giacomelli R, Fontana L, Perricone R. Anti-thyroid antibodies and antiphospholipid syndrome: evidence of reduced fecundity and of poor pregnancy outcome in recurrent spontaneous aborters. *American Journal Reproduction Immunology* 2004;52(4):263–266.

[20] Bussen S, Steck T. Thyroid autoantibodies in euthyroid non-pregnant women with recurrent spontaneous abortions. *Human Reproduction* 1995; 10(11): 2938-2940.

[21] Rushworth F. H, Backos M, Rai R, Chilcott I. T, Baxter N, Regan L. Prospective pregnancy outcome in untreated recurrent miscarriers with thyroid autoantibodies. *Human Reproduction* 2000; 15(7):1637–1639.

[22] Esplin M. S, Branch D. W, Silver R, Stagnaro-Green A. Thyroid autoantibodies are not associated with recurrent pregnancy loss. *American Journal of Obstetrics Gynecology* 1998; 179(6Pt 1):1583–1586.

[23] Negro R, Formoso G, Mangieri T, Pezzarossa A, Dazzi D, Hassan H. Levothyroxine treatment in euthyroid pregnant women with autoimmune thyroid disease: effects on obstetrical complications. *Journal Clinical Endocrinology Metabolism* 2006; 91(7): 2587–2591.

[24] Pearce E. N, Farwell A. P, Braverman L. E. Thyroiditis. *New England Journal of Medicine* 2003; 348(26):2646–2655.

[25] Li Y, Shan Z, Teng W, Yu X, Li Y, Fan C, Teng X, Guo R, Wang H, Li J, Chen Y, Wang W, Chawinga M, Zhang L, Yang L, Zhao Y, Hua T. Abnormalities of maternal thyroid function during pregnancy affect neuropsychological development of their children at 25-30 months. *Clinical Endocrinology* (Oxf) 2010; 72(6):825-829.

In: Hypothyroidism
Editors: A. O'Neill and M. R. Quinn
ISBN: 978-1-62618-872-3

Chapter IV

Hypothyroidism and Desire of Pregnancy: The Education of the Women of Childbearing Age Is Essential!

H. Iraqi,[*] I. Elwadeh and A. Chraibi
Mohammed V University, Souissi, Rabat, Morocco

Abstract

Thyroid hypofunction in pregnancy is associated with either overt or subclinical hypothyroidism. Many studies reported a link between hypothyroidism and infertility as well as with a high rate of spontaneous miscarriages. These pregnancies are though very precious for the patients.

Woman of childbearing age must then be aware of the necessity of an adapted treatment and of a close monitoring in case of a possible pregnancy as well as of risks for herself and for the newborn child.

Once the diagnosis is done, the treatment with oral LT4 is very simple. The monitoring will be made every 2 months (at least) to adapt the treatment to the objectives of TSH which are different from the common population.

[*] Hinde Iraqi. E-mail: hinde_iraqi@hotmail.com.

After a short case report of 15 women of childbearing age followed for hypothyroidism from january to February 2009, we decided to educate all the women of childbearing age because even treated appropriately with oral LT4, they were not sensitized to the necessity of increasing the dose and the follow up in case of pregnancy!

We believe that preconceptional counseling is very important and could improve the management of these very precious pregnancies. In practice, if the hypothyroidism is known, and if a pregnancy is wished, it is necessary to insure a hormonal balance before the conception. We advise to tell the patient they should increase their dose of oral LT4 by 25% to 30%.

Short Communication

Introduction

Thyroid hypofunction in pregnancy is a common situation :it is estimated that 0.3%–0.5% of healthy non pregnant women of childbearing age would, after having thyroid function tests be classified as having overt hypothyroidism (OH), while 2%–2.5% of them would be classified as having subclinical hypothyroidism (SCH). OH is defined as an elevated TSH (>2.5 mIU/L) in conjunction with a decreased FT4 concentration. Women with TSH levels of 10.0 mIU/L or above, irrespective of their FT4 levels, are also considered to have OH. SCH is defined as a serum TSH between 2.5 and 10 mIU/L with a normal FT4 concentration [1-3]. The management of pregnant women with OH is important for themselves and for the fetal health. Appropriateness of tracking pre and postconception maternal thyroid disorders is still discussed. It is recommended in women with personal or familial past history of thyroid diseases; and in women with infertility [4].

Several investigations report a link between hypothyroidism and infertility as well as with a high rate of spontaneous miscarriages [3, 5]. Moreover, thyroidian hormones are mandatory for fetal development especially at the level of brain structures. Any shortage of thyroidian hormone can severely and irreversibly alter neurological development [6]. These pregnancies are though very precious for the patients.

The recommended treatment of maternal hypothyroidism is administration of oral LT4. Other thyroid preparations such as T3 or desiccated thyroid should not be preferred for women of childbearing age who are planning a pregnancy. Women with known hypothyroidism treated with oral LT4 who are newly pregnant should increase their dose of oral LT4 by 25% to 30% and visit their physician promptly. Pregnant women who are positive for TPOAb and have SCH should be treated with LT4. This is a particular situation with no disease but necessity to treat during pregnancy [3]. Preconceptional counseling is though very important is these cases. Women using these drugs must know about the need to change them in case of pregnancy. It is also recommended that all treated hypothyroid women who are planning pregnancy (currently receiving LT4) optimize thyroid status preconception by adjusting their dose (by their physician) in order to optimize serum TSH values to <2.5 mIU/L. If not, the LT4 adjustment should be done as soon as possible after pregnancy is confirmed. Maternal thyroid function tests (FT4 and TSH) should be monitored every 4 to 6 weeks during the first half of pregnancy and then checked at least once between 26 and 32 weeks gestation. The goal is to normalize maternal serum TSH values within the trimester-specific pregnancy reference range (first trimester, 0.1–2.5 mIU/L; second trimester, 0.2–3.0 mIU/L; third trimester, 0.3–3.0 mIU/L) [3].

After a short case report of 15 women of childbearing age followed for hypothyroidism from january to February 2OO9, we decided to educate all the women of childbearing age in our clinic. Our patients were treated appropriately with oral LT4, but they did not know about changes of the doses in case of pregnancy and did not consult their physician promptly! In fact, a patient treated for hypothyroidism with an adequate replacement dose should do a periodic TSH measurement every 6 to 12 months [7]. Woman of childbearing age must then be aware of the necessity of an adapted treatment and of a close monitoring in case of a possible pregnancy as well as of risks for herself and for the newborn child. They would then consult their physician to have the recommended follow up.

A special interest is important for women who have a past history of Graves' disease treated by radioiodine therapy or surgical: a maternal serum determination of Thyroid Stimulating Hormone Receptor Antibody (TRAb) should be done at 20–24 weeks gestation. These autoantibodies cross the placenta and can cause fetal and neonatal thyroid dysfunction even when the mother herself is in a euthyroid condition. The important concern here is that fetal and neonatal hyperthyroidism may still occur. Fetal surveillance with serial ultrasounds should be performed in women with TRAb levels greater than three times the upper limit of normal. A consultation with an experienced obstetrician or maternal–fetal medicine specialist is always necessary [3, 8]. Following delivery, the patient must have their prescription of LT4 reduced to the preconception's dose. Additional TSH testing should be performed at approximately 6 weeks postpartum [3].

Preconceptional counseling is here very important. We believe that counseling about the effects of the disease on maternal health and on fetal well-being could improve the management of these very precious pregnancies.

Conclusion

In practice, we are informing

- every women of childbearing age followed for hypothyroidism that it is necessary to insure a hormonal balance before the conception, so they should increase their dose of oral LT4 by 25% to 30% as soon as the diagnosis of pregnancy is known, and to visit their physician.
- and women who have a past history of Graves' disease treated by radioiodine therapy or surgical who are considered as "cured for their disease" to visit their physician in case of pregnancy whatever are their thyroid status in order to check for the TRAb.
- Following delivery, they have the prescription to reduce the oral LT4 to the preconception dose.
- Because 8 among the 15 women of childbearing age we interviewed thought the breastfeeding is contraindicated with LT4, we also insist on the security of the drug in that situation [3].

References

[1] Glinoer, D. The regulation of thyroid function in pregnancy: pathways of endocrine adaptation from physiology to pathology. *Endocr. Rev.* 1997; 18: 404-33.

[2] Mandel, S. J. Hypothyroidism and chronic auto-immune thyroiditis in the pregnant state: maternal aspects. *Best Pract. Res. Clin. Endocrinol. Metab.* 2004; 18: 213–24.

[3] Stagnaro-Green, A., Abalovich, M., Alexander, E., et al. American thyroid association taskforce on thyroid disease during pregnancy and postpartum. Guidelines of the American thyroid association for the

diagnosis and management of thyroid disease during pregnancy and postpartum. *Thyroid*. 2011;21(10):1081–1125.

[4] Glinoer, D. The regulation of thyroid function during normal pregnancy: importance of the iodine nutrition status. *Best Pract. Res. Clin. Endocrinol. Metab.* 2004;18:133–51

[5] Ashoor, G., Maiz, N., Rotas, M., Jawdat, F., Nicolaides, K. H 2010 Maternal thyroid function at 11 to 13 weeks of gestation and subsequent fetal death. *Thyroid* 20:989–993.

[6] Morreale De Escobar, G., Obregon, M. J., Escobar Del Rey, F. Maternal thyroid hormone early in pregnancy and fetal brain development. *Best Pract. Res. Clin. Endocrinol. Metab.* 2004;18:225–48.

[7] Garber, J. R., Cobin, R. H., Gharib, H., et al. Clinical Practice Guidelines for Hypothyroidism in Adults: Co-sponsored by American Association of Clinical Endocrinologists and the American Thyroid Association. *Endocr. Pract.* 2012 Sep. 11:1-207.

[8] Laurberg, P., Nygaard, B., Glinoer, D., Grussendorf, M., Orgiazzi, J.: Guidelines for TSH-receptor antibody measurements in pregnancy: results of an evidence-based symposium organized by the European Thyroid Association. *Eur. J. Endocrinol.* 139, 584–590 (1998).

Index

N

O

P

R

S

V

W